Misconception

Families in Focus

Series Editors
Anita Ilta Garey, University of Connecticut
Naomi R. Gerstel, University of Massachusetts, Amherst
Karen V. Hansen, Brandeis University
Rosanna Hertz, Wellesley College
Margaret K. Nelson, Middlebury College

Katie L. Acosta, *Amigas y Amantes: Sexually Nonconforming Latinas Negotiate Family*
Anita Ilta Garey and Karen V. Hansen, eds., *At the Heart of Work and Family: Engaging the Ideas of Arlie Hochschild*
Katrina Kimport, *Queering Marriage: Challenging Family Formation in the United States*
Mary Ann Mason, Nicholas H. Wolfinger, and Marc Goulden, *Do Babies Matter? Gender and Family in the Ivory Tower*
Jamie L. Mullaney and Janet Hinson Shope, *Paid to Party: Working Time and Emotion in Direct Home Sales*
Markella B. Rutherford, *Adult Supervision Required: Private Freedom and Public Constraints for Parents and Children*
Barbara Wells, *Daughters and Granddaughters of Farmworkers: Emerging from the Long Shadow of Farm Labor*

Misconception

· ·

Social Class and Infertility in America

ANN V. BELL

Rutgers University Press

New Brunswick, New Jersey, and London

Library of Congress Cataloging-in-Publication Data
Bell, Ann V., 1980–
    Misconception : social class and infertility in America / Ann V. Bell.
        pages cm. — (Families in focus)
    Includes bibliographical references and index.
    ISBN 978–0–8135–6480–7 (hardcover : alk. paper) — ISBN 978–0–8135–6479–1
(pbk. : alk. paper) — ISBN 978–0–8135–6481–4 (e-book)
    1. Infertility, Female—United States. 2. Fertility, Human—United States. 3. Poor
women—United States. 4. Social classes—United States. I. Title.
    RG201.B37 2014
    618.1'7806—dc23   2013046600

A British Cataloging-in-Publication record for this book is available from the
British Library.

Visit our website: http://rutgerspress.rutgers.edu

Manufactured in the United States of America

For Tony

Contents

Acknowledgments

Although there is only one name on the cover of this book, it was entirely a team effort, impossible without the support of numerous players. Thanks to each of you from the bottom of my heart.

Rutgers University Press, particularly Peter Mickulas, has been amazing. You made a difficult process easy and enjoyable. I owe a very special thank you to the editors of the Family in Focus series. Rosanna Hertz got the ball rolling, and Peggy Nelson provided invaluable thoughtful feedback that improved the manuscript immensely.

Without the encouragement, mentoring and support from my graduate advisors, Renee Anspach and Karin Martin, this book would still be just an idea. Renee took the time to help me improve my writing through line-by-line edits and frank, but necessary, constructive criticism. Her knowledge of the field and the breadth and depth of her network and references are impressive and contributed much to the manuscript. I owe a very special thank you to Karin. I call her my "guardian angel": as my undergraduate advisor she developed my interest in sociology, and as my graduate mentor she guided my research. I would not be where I am professionally without her guidance and assistance. I only hope to be half the scholars, mentors, and teachers that Karin and Renee were and are to me.

I would not be where I am today without the incredible love and support from my family. Thank you, Dad, for teaching me how to think critically and reminding me that even Mickey Mantle strikes out sometimes. Thank you, Mom, for always being there to listen and always knowing what to say.

I could not have written this book without the bravery and willingness of the participants to come forward and share their stories. Thank you to the sixty-three women I interviewed. I only hope that I did justice to your experiences and that change may happen because of them.

I have saved my most generous thank you to the end. Thank you for everything, Tony. From constant words of encouragement, to posting flyers, to driving to interviews, to making late dinners, to listening to my brainstorming, and to giving up so much to support me, I thank you and am forever indebted.

In addition, I owe this project thanks for revealing to me the fragility of reproduction. If it were not for my research, I would perhaps not have the most precious people in my life, Abigail and Fiona. Thank you both for showing me what is important in life and for making my life complete.

Misconception

Introduction

· ·

Conceiving Infertility

When I met Angie, a black, homeless, twenty-five-year-old, she was desperately yearning for a child. She told me she wanted a child so that she could "receive love," something that was missing from her own upbringing. Angie had tried to become pregnant through unprotected intercourse for nearly eight years before realizing that something might be "wrong." Her childlessness made her feel "abnormal" among her peers because most of them already had several children. In fact, Angie did not know anyone who had difficulty with childbearing. Although marriage is not important to her, the lack of a commitment made her fearful that her partners would leave her once they discovered her childbearing difficulties so she did not tell them of her troubles. Additionally, because she had no health insurance and because of her negative experiences with physicians, she did not seek medical care. Ultimately, Angie, accustomed to not getting everything she wanted in life, was forced to cope with her infertility and primarily sought solace through prayer.

Sarah, a white, upper-middle-class, thirty-three-year-old, also told me about her childbearing difficulties. After completing college, establishing a career, and getting married, Sarah decided it was time to have a child. But after just six months of trying with temperature taking and ovulation kits, she began to worry about why she was not conceiving. She described her husband as her strongest support system and said talking to her friends was her "therapy" for getting through her reproductive troubles. Several of Sarah's peers who delayed childbearing to focus on their careers were still childless so Sarah felt like she "fit in." Upon recognizing her difficulties, Sarah immediately went to the doctor and began fertility treatments. She complemented the medicine with weekly acupuncture and massage appointments. If her current medications failed to result in pregnancy, Sarah planned to continue medical procedures "as the doctor orders," including intrauterine inseminations (IUIs) and in vitro fertilizations (IVFs). She could not imagine a life without children. Motherhood was something she had always wanted, and this situation presented one of the few occasions in her life when things had not gone according to plan.

Both Sarah and Angie described living with infertility, yet they experienced it in two very different ways. Only Sarah's story, however, and stories like it have been told. Infertility is stereotypically depicted as a white, wealthy woman's issue, shaped by media images of celebrities receiving IVFs and reality shows highlighting the lives of families with sets of multiples (Throsby 2004). But in reality, poor women and women of color have equivalent, if not slightly higher, rates of infertility than their wealthier counterparts (Chandra, Copen, and Stephen 2013; Marsh and Ronner 1996).[1] Marginalized women's stories of infertility have been silenced, however, by social misconceptions about race, class, reproduction, and fertility. The media, medical texts, and social policies have continuously lauded the childbearing practices of higher-class, white women. Policies have encouraged affluent women to have children, even at times prohibiting such women from having abortions (Gordon 2002). In contrast, the fertility and reproductive practices of economically disadvantaged women and women of color have been criticized; namely, the belief persists that poor women have too many children. By focusing on their "hyperfertility," policies and popular culture have overshadowed the presence of infertility among marginalized women (Cussins 1998).

Not only do political and popular cultures promulgate a particular image of *who* is infertile, but they also perpetuate a particular understanding of *what* infertility is (Greil, McQuillan, and Slauson-Blevins 2011). Infertility is not only stereotyped as affecting affluent, white women, but it is also viewed as a health issue requiring medical treatment (Becker and Nachtigall 1992). The medicalization of infertility, or its transformation from a natural life event into a problem that requires medical treatment, developed with the advent of assisted reproductive technologies (ARTs) in the late 1970s and early 1980s. Since the birth of Louise Brown, the first baby born from IVF, ARTs and other fertility treatments have proliferated, making infertility synonymous with its medical treatment (Wilcox and Mosher 1993). Media representations of infertility reinforce such depictions, highlighting ARTs as the acceptable solution. For instance, in recent years the *New York Times* published articles headlined "Million Dollar Babies," "Lessons from the Test Tube," "The Gift of Life, and Its Price"; all of these focus on the medical treatment of infertility, primarily its high cost and ethical implications. Media critics argue that IVF needs to be made more widely available, but they rarely question whether it is the best solution for infertility (De Lacey 2002).

Both stereotypes, depicting who is infertile and what infertility is, make the infertility experiences of marginalized women, like Angie, invisible (Inhorn, Ceballo, and Nachtigall 2009). Women of low socioeconomic status (SES) cannot afford medical treatments for infertility, and, along with women of color, they do not fit the typical image of the "infertile woman." Research also contributes to their exclusion from our understanding of infertility. Understandably, for convenience, most infertility studies recruit participants from medical clinics (Greil, Slauson-Blevins, and McQuillan 2010). In so doing, however, the academic portrayal concentrates on the medical dimensions of infertility and examines those who are lucky enough to receive medical care: typically white, higher-class women. There is virtually no research on poor and working-class women's experiences of infertility or the lived experience of infertility outside the doctor's office (Culley 2009).

My goal in this book is to center rather than marginalize the infertility experiences of women of low SES. By bringing their stories to light and comparing them to the white women of high SES we typically associate with infertility, the book begins to break down the stereotypes of infertility and show how such depictions consequently shape women's infertility experiences. Comparing the experiences of women of different races and classes reveals how race, class, and gender intersect in the institutions of motherhood and medicine. As I argue, infertility is a social process, influenced by class- and race-based ideas around reproduction, motherhood, family, and health. These ideas shape our understanding of who is infertile and what infertility is.

Who Is Infertile: The Construction
of the "Good" and "Bad" Mother

Social conceptions of motherhood have long constructed the role of mother as universal, stable, and essential to women's nature. According to the "motherhood mandate," womanhood equates with motherhood, and motherhood is therefore expected of all women (Russo 1976). In turn, childlessness is viewed as abnormal. The current ideology around mothering, however, known as "intensive mothering," complicates the motherhood mandate (Hays 1996). It outlines *who* should mother as well as *how* one should mother according to idealized family norms. Intensive mothering is based upon a white, middle-class, heterosexual gold standard to which other mothers are compared. According to this standard, good mothers are those self-sacrificing and child-centered women who can afford to stay home with their children. Women unable to fulfill this ideal are marginalized and systematically devalued (Connolly 2000; McCormack 2005).

The intersection of intensive mothering with the motherhood mandate poses a problem for women who cannot adhere to one or both of these ideals. Poor and working-class women experiencing infertility form one such group: not only are they childless and therefore unable to fulfill the motherhood mandate, but they are also unable to meet the physical, emotional, and financial demands of intensive mothering.

Unlike their wealthier counterparts, women of low SES are constructed as bad mothers. They are expected to fulfill middle-class standards of motherhood even though they lack the social and economic resources to do so (Baker and Carson 1999; McCormack 2005). Nowhere are these contradictions more apparent than in the case of the welfare mother. As poor women, welfare recipients are expected (and forced) to look for work to overcome their impoverished state. As mothers, however, the notion of intensive mothering expects them to focus exclusively on mothering (Hays 1996). Thus, not only are increased and contradictory demands placed upon women of low SES, but they are also set up for failure according to social expectations of good mothering (Solinger 2013).

Media commentators and politicians often overlook this predicament when they focus exclusively on poor and working-class mothers' parenting and call it inadequate, while ignoring the actual context of their lives. Women deemed bad mothers are criticized as individuals, and their parenting style is attributed to their personal failings, thereby shifting focus away from how such a label is situated in notions of race and class. Bad mothers are blamed for irresponsibility, lack of control, and poor decision making, while structural factors such as poverty, lack of resources, and limited support are disregarded (Abramovitz 1995; Collins 1994).

The ideas of the good mother and the bad mother, based on a stratified system of reproduction in which fertility is differently valued according to an individual's race and class, play out in policies and practices around fertility (Colen 1986; Greil et al. 2011b; Roberts 1997). The eugenics movement in the first half of the century, the forced sterilization abuses of the 1960s and 1970s, and federally funded family planning programs that began in the 1970s all reinforced the binary understanding of good mother versus bad mother (King and Meyer 1997; Steinberg 1997). These programs attempted to reduce the reproduction of those deemed unfit or abnormal—often members of marginalized groups, such as poor women and women of color. These movements also affected white women of high SES who were subject to pronatalist policies and therefore unable to access ways to limit their reproduction (Glenn 1994). After the Supreme Court decision in *Roe v. Wade,* abortion came under the control of medicine rather than individual women. Acting in concert with reproductive norms, physicians, as gatekeepers to abortions, encouraged and discouraged the procedure along socioeconomic lines. In turn, access to abortions ironically remained limited for higher-class women once abortion was legalized (Gordon 2002).

Current reproductive benefits around infertility reflect such class- and race-based ideas (Solinger 2013). Insurance coverage of infertility treatments is implicitly grounded in the logic developed in the eugenic period: treating the infertility of the affluent and controlling the fertility of the poor (King and Meyer 1997; Steinberg 1997). As of 2013, fourteen states have laws that require private insurers to fully cover, partially cover, or offer to cover some form of infertility diagnosis and treatment (American Society for Reproductive Medicine 2013a).[2] An unequal distribution of reproductive benefits, however, remains, based on social class. In Illinois, for example, the state mandates that employer-based insurers cover infertility treatment, yet poor women on Medicaid do not receive such benefits. In contrast, Medicaid mandates contraceptive coverage for its recipients, yet the same is not true for women with private, employer-based insurance policies. This "dualistic natalist policy" discourages births among women of low SES and encourages them among women of higher classes (King and Meyer 1997).

What Infertility Is: The Medicalization
of Infertility and Its Consequences

Today, it is hard to imagine thinking about infertility without also think-ing about its medical treatment, but the medicalization of infertility is a relatively recent phenomenon. Prior to the 1970s and the proliferation of ARTs, infertility was considered one of life's unfortunate events that could be resolved through either adoption or the acceptance of childlessness (Becker and Nachtigall 1992). In fact, there was *resistance* to treating infer-tility medically. A 1969 Harris poll revealed that the majority of Americans believed IVF was "against God's will," and in 1972 the American Medical Association even encouraged a moratorium on all IVF research. The turn-ing point came in 1978, with the birth of the first "test tube baby," Lou-ise Brown, in Great Britain. The media frenzy that followed, including a reported half a million dollars to the Browns for rights to the story, ignited much excitement around medicine's role in infertility. Just one month after Brown's birth, a new survey revealed that more than 60 percent of Ameri-cans now supported IVF and would consider doing it themselves. And one year later, in 1979, the National Institutes of Health granted federal fund-ing for IVF research.

These shifts in attitudes toward reproductive technology, combined with the increasing number of women entering the workforce and delay-ing childbearing, led to a perfect storm in the late 1970s that proliferated the medical treatment of infertility and the development of its specialty, reproductive endocrinology (Marsh and Ronner 1996). The rest is history. Between 1968 and 1984, medical visits for infertility tripled from 600,000 to 1.6 million (Greil 1991). More recently, between 1995 and 2002, the use of ARTs doubled from nearly 60,000 cycles in 1995 to approximately 116,000 cycles only seven years later (Jain 2006).[3] And the numbers con-tinue to rise, with more than 160,000 cycles conducted in 2011 (Centers for Disease Control and Prevention 2013a).

ARTs, presented as a triumph in the media and by physicians, created the impression that infertility is a disease that could be cured, and women could, for the first time, "choose" to become biological parents. Nursing scholar Margarete Sandelowski (1993, 45) insightfully notes that "infertil-ity has only recently come to mean the potential to have a child of one's own, rather than merely the incapacity to have a child on one's own." In other words, medically treating infertility reinvented the condition as an indeterminate, liminal state of not *yet* pregnant, thereby making the mandate of motherhood all the more prominent (Greil 1991). Additionally, with the development of reproductive technologies, choosing to have a child, when to have a child, and how to have a child have become commonplace discussions among prospective parents. Individuals increasingly see reproduction as more of a choice, which makes infertility seem all the more volitional (Sandelowski 1990).

For the vast majority of women, however, the idea that we have conquered infertility is illusory. Infertility treatments are expensive—the average cost of one cycle of IVF is $12,400—and many women undergo more than one round of treatment (American Society for Reproductive Medicine 2013b). As previously noted, only a few states require private insurance coverage for infertility care, and Medicaid does not cover any treatment. These policies withhold the choice from poor women, and ART is beyond the reach of even some middle-class women. According to the most recent National Survey of Family Growth (NSFG), among women experiencing reproductive problems, only 5 percent with less than a college education received ART compared to nearly 20 percent with at least a bachelor's degree (Chandra, Stephen, and King 2013). In other words, the medicalization of infertility reinforces the stratified system of reproduction by providing the option of reproduction to some groups and not to others. In turn, women of low SES are confronted with a double stigma: they are not socially recognized as mothers due to their infertility, but they are additionally shunned for their desires to be mothers in the first place (Spar 2006). Medicalizing infertility does not unite women around the commonality of medicine (or motherhood); instead, it perpetuates the differences between them (Litt 1997).

Even for the few women who can afford to pay out-of-pocket for infertility treatments, such treatments are not always successful: in 2010, only 30 percent of ART cycles resulted in a live birth—a 70 percent failure rate (Centers for Disease Control and Prevention 2013b).[4] The fact that women are willing to undergo costly, protracted treatment for a mere possibility of success attests to the high value we place on biological kinship; it also reveals the extent of our faith in medicine (Franklin 2013). In turn, the medicalization of infertility makes it less likely that affluent women will pursue other ways (for example, adoption or foster care) of fulfilling the motherhood mandate (Quiroga 2007).

The emphasis placed on biological kinship is the primary reason infertility treatments even exist. The absence of a desired condition, having a biological child, not the pathological condition, such as hyperprolactinemia (high levels of prolactin in the blood), causes individuals to seek medical care for infertility. Infertility does not require a cure in order to be considered healthy. Indeed, treatments do not target the etiologic factors of infertility; instead, they circumvent those factors in an attempt to achieve the desired outcome, a biological child (Sandelowski 1990). Only one treatment, tubal surgery, actually attempts to cure infertility. All other treatments aim at conceiving a biological child, but individuals remain infertile after that is accomplished. In other words, medical interventions cure biological childlessness, not infertility per se (Evans 1995; Sandelowski 1993). In defining it as a physiological state, however, medical texts and physicians make infertility seem objective and rooted in biology; thus, its basis in social norms is overlooked (Greil 1991; Greil 1997; Scritchfield 1989).

Similar to circumstances that occurred prior to the development of reproductive technologies, women of low SES, unable to access infertility treatments, are forced to cope with the condition as a part of life, but the difference now is that they are aware of potential, yet unattainable, remedies to their difficulties. In other words, they are "outsiders-within" the context of (medicalized) infertility (Collins 1994). They are able to reflect on both the dominant and the subordinate experiences of infertility. Economically disadvantaged women, having unique insight to the stratified system of reproduction, thus expose infertility as a social process.

About This Study

With this premise of inequality and diversity in mind, I set out to investigate how and why the social construction of infertility—or who we typically think of as infertile and what we typically think of as infertility—shapes the infertility experiences of women of diverse social classes. To do so, I conducted fifty-eight in-depth interviews with women who were between the ages of eighteen and forty-four and had been involuntarily childless for at least twelve months due to the inability to become pregnant or carry a child to term (medical definition for infertility). To participate in the study, the women could have experienced involuntary childlessness at any point in their lives. This means that, for some of the participants (n=eight), infertility is a thing of the past as they currently have children or are no longer *involuntarily* childless because they have "moved on" in life. Having such open eligibility criteria allowed me to interview the number of participants needed for the study, given the limited number of women willing to talk about their childbearing difficulties.[5] The majority of participants (n=fifty) were still experiencing infertility during the research, as most did not have children and/or were still struggling with their childbearing pursuits. Additionally, the maximum age for participating was forty-four years old, which means that infertility, if a thing of the past, is a relatively recent occurrence because women's childbearing years are limited.[6]

As I explain further in the appendix, I divided the women into two socioeconomic groups—low SES and high SES. I based these groupings on theoretical and empirical divisions. I primarily used income to determine the categorization of participants, but ultimately I used a conglomeration of factors, including the participant's occupation, education, parents' education, and subjective assessment of income adequacy. Two-thirds of the participants were white women and black women of low SES, and the remaining one-third were white women of high SES. These three particular groupings happened both purposefully and accidentally. I purposefully oversampled women of low SES for several reasons. First, my primary concern in this study was to better understand how class shapes the experience of infertility because that is the dimension by which women are *explicitly* excluded from receiving medical treatment for their infertility. Second, the scant research that has been done on the experiences of infertility among diverse women examines its racial dimensions, but its basis in economics has been less explored. Third, I needed to listen to the experiences of economically marginalized women, not only to bring their silenced stories to light but also because their experiences, as outsiders-within the healthcare system, exposed nuances in higher-class women's infertility journeys that affluent women, alone, could not comprehend.

In spite of my intended research design, this study is composed of three rather than four groups. Initially I set out to have four groups: the three included in this study as well as black women of high SES. Despite extensive efforts to recruit such participants, in the end I was only able to interview three women fitting that category, not enough for conclusive, rigorous comparison. I believe this occurred for several reasons. First, the participants in the study reflect the general demographics of southeastern Michigan, the area in which I recruited—there are few affluent, black women in the region. Second, wealthy black women may be less willing to participate in research because their infertility experiences are absent from mainstream discourse; thus, they feel alone and silenced (Ceballo 1999). Although future work needs to be done on black women of high SES, for this study, focusing on the comparisons between white women and black women of low SES and white women of high SES makes theoretical and empirical sense. Because I began the study primarily interested in how mainstream ideas about infertility affect its experience, comparing women excluded from those narratives (women of low SES) to women enmeshed within them (*white* women of high SES) is appropriate. Additionally, because my main focus is on class differences in infertility, it makes sense to oversample women of low SES and compare them to women of high SES, generally, regardless of race. The racial comparison within the low SES groups, however, allowed me to achieve a more nuanced analysis that did not overgeneralize my findings to all women in a certain class. (See the appendix for a more detailed explanation of my sample and methods.)

As you read the following pages, you will note significant differences in infertility experiences between the socioeconomic groups. I am confident that such differences are owing to class rather than other characteristics, such as marital status and age, which also differed among women. For instance, through comparative analysis I found that differences in the ways women "tried" to become pregnant did not vary by marital status, but they did differ by SES status. Of course, such characteristic differences by class *are* themselves part and parcel of the classed experiences (Jones and Hunter 1996). Women of low SES do, on average, have children at younger ages and marry less frequently (McMahon 1995). I explore how those practices play out and shape experiences of infertility throughout the book. I caution readers, however, to avoid placing their own stereotypes on the participants in this study. For example, not all women of high SES were infertile because they delayed childbearing. Indeed, this was the explicit case for only one of the high SES participants, as the majority of women of high SES were under age thirty-five. Additionally, age-related infertility was present for two of the low SES participants.

About This Book

Conducting in-depth interviews allowed me to gain comprehensive, nuanced insight into the *lived experiences* of infertility. Through the women's stories, I traced the entire infertility experience from before the women realized they had childbearing difficulties to how they became aware of and coped with the problem and how they planned for the future. In the book I walk through their journeys chronologically. In chapter 1 I ask the basic question of why the women want to mother in the first place. I follow in chapter 2 by examining how the women negotiate such maternal desires in a context that portrays them as fit or unfit for the motherhood role. I continue to explore life before infertility in chapter 3 by comparing various ways women try to become pregnant. Subsequently, in chapter 4 I thoroughly discuss what it is like for them to live with infertility, particularly in their social environments. I begin to elucidate life after infertility in chapter 5 by exploring how the women sought medical and nonmedical solutions to the problem. In chapter 6 I then ask how the women cope with infertility and how they envision their futures. Finally, in my conclusion I revisit the significance of the findings and particularly discuss their policy implications.

The findings that I present in this book focus on how class shapes the experience of infertility. Yet, the racial diversity of the women of low SES allowed me to explore race as well. I found class to be more salient than race in shaping experiences of infertility, a finding similar to those of other researchers examining the class and race dynamics of family processes (for example, Edin and Kefalas 2005; Lareau 2003). Women of low SES in this study reported similar experiences, regardless of their race. Yet, when comparing the stories told by women of high SES with those told by women of low SES the differences were significant. When differences between races do arise, however, I both highlight them in the text and summarize them in the conclusion.

Exploring experiences of infertility among a diverse group of women not only challenges our stereotypical notion of who is infertile but also exposes differences and similarities in experiences of infertility that arise out of varying social locations. In doing so, this study reveals infertility as a social process, one rooted in social norms and shaped by social context, rather than merely a single, uniform, objective medical experience (Greil, Slauson-Blevins, and McQuillan 2010). Angie and Sarah both experienced infertility, yet their experiences differed dramatically. The following chapters, exploring how and why such differences exist, ultimately reveal the depth and complexity of infertility experiences, experiences that are rooted in class- and race-based ideas about family, motherhood, health, and reproduction.

1

"That's What I'm Supposed to Be"

● ●

Why Women Want to Mother

After I got a little wilder and when I got a little older, I thought definitely [motherhood] would slow me down. And people would tell me that. My friends and acquaintances, they'd say, "You just need a baby. You'll slow down."
—Candace, black woman of low SES

I always thought you would just grow up and get married and, you know, you go to college and after you go to college, you get married. And then you have kids. That's what's supposed to happen.
—Becca, white woman of high SES

Why do women want to mother? It seems like a simple question, yet few researchers have looked for the answer. In studying infertility, asking such a question seemed like an intuitive place for me to start because implicit in the very definition of infertility is intentionality of pregnancy: a woman must want or "try" to become pregnant in order to recognize her inability to conceive. So, I wondered, why did the women want to mother in the first place? As the findings demonstrate, this simple question begs a not-so-simple answer.

Until the 1980s, sociologists failed to inquire about why women want to mother. One explanation for this silence may be the deeply embedded, taken-for-granted "motherhood mandate." The answer was simply assumed; for a woman, being a mother is not a choice; womanhood equals motherhood (Russo 1976). The motherhood literature reified this assumption through its failure to ask why women would strive to attain such a role. By not questioning the assumption, research reinforces the idea that motherhood is an innate desire for all women, strictly a gendered phenomenon, unrelated to race or class.

Despite its paucity, a few researchers have broached the topic of women's mothering motivations. Nancy Chodorow's landmark work *The Reproduction of Mothering* (1978) was one of the first to inquire about why women want to mother. Chodorow concludes that motherhood is reproduced through the gendered structure of parenting. The primary characteristics of mothering, such as caretaking and nurturance, develop in a woman's personality as a result of her identification with and attachment to her own mother. In this psychoanalytic account, women pursue mothering to enact and to regain those feelings that have become a part of them. In a similar yet different vein, through her theory of maternal thinking philosopher Sarah Ruddick (1989) studies why women mother. Unlike Chodorow's psychoanalytic approach, which understands mothering as developing within an individual's psyche, Ruddick argues that those characteristics are products of maternal practice, or the "doing" of mothering. Although both studies contribute much to our understanding of motherhood, they universalize mothering desires and fail to examine how such motivations may differ among women.

Studies that do examine diversity in mothering typically focus on negative effects of race and class (for example, welfare moms), relate the demographics to policy issues, or include race and class to compare mothering practices rather than motivations (for example, Lareau 2003). For instance, sociologists Kathryn Edin and Maria Kefalas (2005) conducted one of the few studies that examines why marginalized women want to mother, yet such an analysis was secondary to their primary inquiry of why poor women do not marry before having children. Their research focused on policy rather than theory. Additionally, while their study provides excellent insight into why poor women desire motherhood, it did not compare such desires among women of different races or social classes and is thus unable to explore why or how different contexts and norms lead to different mothering ideals.

As the women in this book demonstrate, however, there are striking class differences in why women want to mother. Women of low SES desire motherhood for the individual advantages they will gain from having a baby so their motivations are centered around the effects of having a child; women of high SES, however, want to mother not because of what the child will bring to them, but because of the mothering role itself. Higher-class women have internalized mainstream ideas around motherhood, and attaining those social norms motivates their desire to mother. For instance, Becca's epigraph at the chapter opening demonstrates how women of high SES are concerned about fulfilling their class prescriptions of having children at certain stages of their lives. By way of contrast, Candace's quote shows how women of low SES are more concerned about how the baby will change them as individuals. Women of high SES believe you should have a child after achieving adulthood, while women of low SES hope that the child brings about such maturity. Such a distinction leads the women on different journeys to motherhood and thus different experiences of infertility.

These class differences demonstrate that motherhood is more than just a role. Answers to the question of why women want to mother reveal the complexity of motherhood and expose how motherhood intersects with race and class. The diversity of participants allows us to explore how individuals' decisions are influenced by cultural discourses. Put simply, the diversity provides us with an opportunity to discover how women, particularly members of subordinate groups, position themselves vis-à-vis the greater society. Asking why women want to mother among infertile women is especially noteworthy because this group is intentionally trying to mother. This offers a prospective look at mothering, which is rare, particularly among economically disadvantaged women and removes the bias that may ensue when asking women about mothering desires after they have had a child. This approach also allows us to further understand the infertility experience because mothering motivations shape the consequences of infertility (Ulrich and Weatherall 2000).

Why Women Want to Mother: Focusing on the Baby

The United States is a pronatalist culture: policies and practices generally encourage reproduction. In turn, pronatalism perpetuates the notion that "motherhood is the defining element of true womanhood" (Parry 2005a, 338). Such gendered allocation of mothering reduces women to their reproductive capacities. Indeed, womanhood and motherhood are treated as synonymous identities to the extent that mothering is not a choice for women; rather, it is socially mandated. Yet such a motherhood mandate is naturalized and therefore invisible. By being intertwined with a woman's body and her reproduction, most individuals disregard the social, political, and moral aspects of mothering.

The potency and embeddedness of pronatalism and the motherhood mandate, however, are apparent in the participants' mothering motivations. Women of high and low SES share only one response regarding mothering motivations: they want to mother because of an innate desire. Carla, a friendly and motivated black woman of low SES, reflects: "I think like that's what I'm supposed—I'm supposed to be a mother. That's how I look at it. I'm supposed to be— . . . That's just it, you know . . . I had—it was—it was in me to want to be." Similarly, Courtney, a petite white woman of high SES, cannot explain why she wants children because it is an instinctual response: "I just—it's not like I ever thought about it. I just knew I was going to be a mom and it was like inbred in me. I knew—inbred—ingrained. I just—I—I knew it was going to happen." Carla and Courtney internalize the notion that all women mother. They accept the motherhood mandate unquestioningly; they believe that their desires are innate and that they are "supposed" to be mothers.

Given the essential nature of the motherhood mandate, it is not surprising that this theme runs through all the women's accounts of their mothering desires. Yet, beyond the notion that, as a woman, one should mother, stark differences arise among the women's mothering motivations. Because the maternal instinct does not solely arise in biology but in the social and cultural factors surrounding motherhood, a woman's contextual circumstances, such as what social messages are received, play a large role in her decision making around motherhood.

The women of low SES I interviewed focused on the *outcomes* of mothering—the baby and the effects of having a baby. They were *baby*-focused in that all of their mothering desires centered on the child and what he or she would provide to them. The women of low SES rarely discussed the importance of following dominant cultural norms and mandates in their accounts of mothering desires. This view is similar to the findings of Emily Martin (1990) regarding the medicalization of reproduction and Linda Blum (1999) on mainstream practices of infant feeding in which women of marginalized groups were either not conscious of or disregarded the dominant ideals. Working-class black women did not feel guilty about bottle-feeding their children, unlike their white counterparts who were upset about not meeting the norm of breast-feeding. Such findings demonstrate the importance of social location in shaping women's recognition and utilization of cultural norms in their daily lives.

The women of low SES wanted to mother in order to fill a void in their lives. Many women understood that gap as not receiving enough love and attention; therefore, they desired a child, both to give and receive love. As sociologist Martha McMahon (1995) found, many women desire motherhood to escape impoverished, unhealthy situations. Motherhood allows them to find safety and nurturance. When asked why she wanted to mother, Angie, a black woman of low SES, states: "Why actually do I want a baby so bad? I have no idea. But it has been on my mind ever since I was sixteen years old and it's not going to go away until I have a kid. And I—I—I don't know what's wrong with me. I have no idea. Maybe—maybe it's because not enough affection in the family and not enough love. Maybe that's what it is. Maybe I think I can get, you know, break that cycle if I have a kid or something. (Laughs) I have no idea. I have no idea." Angie wants to have a child for what the child will give to her—love—something that she believes was lacking in her own upbringing.

Many women of low SES want children to ensure they have someone to care for them when they are older. Such a desire may reflect both a realization that in their childhood experiences they needed but did not receive care and a fear that such neglect might be replicated when they require caretaking again at an advanced age. Additionally, this reasoning demonstrates the cultural practice of extended kin networks in low-income communities (Stack 1975). Given a lack of institutional and social supports (for example, nursing homes) that are prevalent and accessible in high-income settings, individuals in economically disadvantaged neighborhoods rely on family to fulfill certain needs (Jarrett, Jefferson, and Kelly 2010). Such needs cannot be met unless such a family exists. Moreover, this concern might be particularly acute for poor women because, as women, they are at increased risk for poverty in old age and, as impoverished women, they are more likely to be unmarried without familial support in that capacity (Lee 2009).

Heather, a biracial low SES office assistant, reflects on these concerns: "Well, when I die, I don't want to die alone, whether it's before or after [my husband]. I said, 'But if I'm sick and I'm dying, I want my children and my grandchildren and my family to be there.' And so I guess that's a whole different perspective of having kids because it's having the extended family because my parents will be gone and my sister may or may not still be here but if I'm old and, you know, and dying, I want it to be with family. You know, and just not in a home somewhere." Heather is aware that her nuclear family members, including her parents and siblings, may not be alive when she requires care at an older age. She wants children to meet such a foreseeable need.

In addition to wanting a child in order to receive love and support, women of low SES want to be mothers in order to prove their social worth. Motherhood may be the only way poor and working-class women can achieve fulfillment because they are many times surrounded by poverty, unemployment, crime, and drugs. Rhonda, a homeless white woman of low SES in her mid-forties, reflects: "[A child would be] just something to hang onto, I guess. You know, something to (pauses)—maybe to make my life complete, you know? Or, you know, that we were—to show that I could do something like maybe my life wasn't perfect but I could, you know, reverse the role and (laughs)—it would have been a good thing, too." Similar to Angie, Rhonda hopes that having a baby will "reverse" or "break the cycle" of her life situation.

Candace, a short-haired black woman of low SES, also believes a child will steer her on the right path: "I had a lot of anger. And I had a lot of issues going on inside. . . . [I thought a baby] was going to make everything all right. Because I was going to be able to care for another baby, another child, another person. And I was going to be able to do something good for somebody that was mine."

In addition to "doing something good for somebody" Candace was motivated to mother because of its redemptive characteristics. The "motive of redemptive motherhood" is the belief that having children invokes maturity and reduces irresponsible behaviors, such as partying and drugs (McMahon 1995, 169). Candace demonstrates such reasoning when she told me: "After I got a little wilder and when I got a little older, I thought definitely [motherhood] would slow me down. And people would tell me that. My friends and acquaintances, they'd say, 'You just need a baby. You'll slow down.' Because it—it was this loving girl and environment that was so messed up." Candace was an alcoholic who had been imprisoned numerous times. She hoped that having a baby would "slow her down" and thus resolve the drug and alcohol issues in her life. Viewing motherhood as a symbol of adulthood is the opposite of the higher-class view in which one strives to achieve adulthood prior to becoming a mother.

The mothering motivations mentioned thus far were similar across both white and black women of low SES. A motivation unique to the black participants, however, was the desire to have a child of one's "own." This may stem from the predominance of community mothering in the context of black, low-income women. Driven by cultural practices and need, black women of low SES often share the care of children among extended families and social networks (Blum and Deussen 1996). As "other mothers," these women care for friends' and family members' children as if they were their "own," but at the end of the day they have to "give it back." Doing so can evoke the desire to mother as it did for Roxanne, a black woman of low SES employed part-time at a daycare center: "Because it's like very important to me to like have my own child. Because it's like I can like have my sister's baby or my brother's baby or whoever else's baby but it's like when it's time to give it back, it's like, 'Dang, if this was my own child, I wouldn't have to give it back.'" Roxanne wants a child for herself, one she can call her "own." This response was unique to, but typical of black women of low SES in contrast to their white counterparts. Such a cultural practice causes women to want children not only because it makes them realize the value of permanency in the relationship but also because community mothering makes them feel prepared to take on the challenge of parenting.

Why Women Want to Mother: Focusing on Motherhood

For poor and working-class women, motherhood fills a need absent in other areas of their lives, but for women of high SES, whose basic needs are fulfilled, motherhood serves a different purpose—it allows them to maintain and achieve normality (Hennessy 2009). Mothering desires among women of high SES are centered on the *process* of mothering—its role, attainment, and trajectory. They were *mother*-focused because all their responses centered on motherhood itself. For example, Maureen, a talkative white woman of high SES, wants a child to make her marriage and family more legitimate: "But there's this idea that—that who we are would be more legitimate, you know, that the sense of my husband and I as a family unit would be more legitimate if there were a child in the picture." Maureen has internalized traditional views that the purpose of marriage is for procreation and that families should include children. She desires a child to achieve those ideals and thus achieve legitimacy. Even though Maureen is a heterosexual, middle-class, white, married woman, all dominant-group characteristics, she still does not feel "legitimate" according to social norms. Not being a mother as a married woman makes Maureen the "other" in mainstream understandings of womanhood and thus evokes feelings of illegitimacy.

Contained within these mainstream notions of womanhood is how and when motherhood should be achieved. For women of high SES, a singular, linear life-course trajectory is typical (for example, go to college, get married, have children . . .), whereas women of low SES have more varied trajectories. Many poor and working-class women have children prior to marriage (Edin and Kefalas 2005) or attain a college degree while working later in life (McDonough 1997). But for women of high SES, achieving each stage in life is necessary to maintain normality. Becca, a red-haired white woman of high SES, demonstrates this plan when she states: "I guess I always wanted kids. I always thought you would just grow up and get married and, you know, you go to college and after you go to college, you get married. And then you have kids. That's what's supposed to happen." Becca wants a child because, according to her, that is "what's supposed to happen" at this particular time in her life. To fulfill the prescriptions of her class, having children is the next thing to do. For women of high SES, you should "grow up" prior to becoming a mother. This trajectory differs from the low SES women's desire to mother in order to achieve adulthood. The distinction is time-bound: low SES want to mother so that it brings them maturity; high SES want to achieve maturity before they mother. Women of high and low SES have different life-courses, and those various paths lead them to different reasons for wanting to mother.

Nadia, a serious and direct white woman of high SES, describes the embeddedness of the higher-class trajectory: "Not because—it's because it's like I mean, 'Hey, we're thirty-three.' And you look around and it's like, 'What? Something's missing.' You know, we've been married—we have— long enough that we have had time to do all we wanted to do, you know, together. We have traveled, we have, you know, got—gotten a further level of our—our relationship and it's like, 'Okay, now what?' It just seems like the next step. And it is! It's naturally the next step. I mean it's a birthright, right?" For Nadia, becoming a mother is not only a "birthright" but also the "natural" occurrence after certain life events are achieved. Traveling, an established relationship, and doing "all we wanted to do" was not enough. Unlike women of low SES who did not receive the basic necessities in life and desired children to fulfill those needs, women of high SES such as Nadia, whose basic needs were met, desired children because kids were "missing" from their adherence to ideological notions of womanhood and motherhood.

Two of the high SES participants expressed religious motivation for mothering. Nan believed that being a mother "was a calling as a married couple that . . . God desired for us." Dominant ideology is still apparent within such motivation. Like Maureen's drive for legitimacy, heteronormative definitions of family and views of procreation as the purpose of marriage are implicit in Nan's reasoning.

Adherence to social norms drives the high SES women's motivations for mothering. Because of the uniformity of those norms in higher-class culture, there are far fewer types of responses and variation in reasoning among women of high SES when compared to the answers of women of low SES (Harding 2007). Additionally, the responses of women of high SES compared to those of women of low SES were more vague. Many middle- and upper-class women had difficulty articulating why they wanted to mother. This may be because the reasons women of high SES want to mother are based on dominant ideologies, yet those ideologies are so commonplace that they go unrecognized. Carole, an animated white woman of high SES, did not know why she wanted to be a mother, but she just "always knew [she'd] be a mom." Similarly, Nadia stumbles as she attempts to answer why she wants to be a mother: "Oh, gosh, that's a hard—that's a good, hard question. I guess for me, it's—I mean I have always been rather maternal . . . —I don't know—you learn—you use everything you have learned to help make a life of somebody else better. I don't know. I mean I—that's such a hard way to describe. . . . It's—it's hard. It's hard. It's just something that I have wanted more than anything else. Very strongly."

Understanding why women want to mother sheds light on the various consequences that might ensue should motherhood not be attained. At stake for women of low SES is not fulfilling basic needs. They will need to look elsewhere to receive love, "hope that their nieces remember [them]" when they require care in old age, and redefine what constitutes their "own" children. In contrast, women of high SES will be required to cope with their "otherness." For many of these women, it is the first time they have not achieved a life goal and the first time they find themselves in a subordinate position (with the exception of their status as women). They will need to reevaluate normality and their place in society. All women, regardless of social position, will need to reconstruct their gendered identity. An instinctual, innate desire fails to come to fruition, revealing both the unnaturalness of motherhood and the fragility of reproduction.

2

"I'm Good at the Job"

• • • • • • • • • • • • • • • • • • • •

How Women Achieve
"Good" Motherhood

> And I think good moms are the ones
> that are able to protect their kids from
> bad things happening. And I think good
> moms are there.
> —Lynn, white woman of low SES

> A good mother is somebody who loves
> their children unconditionally and who
> will I mean basically lay down their life
> for their children. . . . Someone who
> is selfless and giving to their children
> makes a good mother. . . . It's just having
> that desire to—to be active and—and—
> and interactive in your child's life.
> —Courtney, white woman of high SES

We see it on a daily basis—the news media criticizing certain types of mothering: mothers who leave their children locked in hot cars, "latch-key" children left alone while their single mothers are at work, teenage parents too immature to raise children, and emotionally damaged children of divorced parents. While these are extreme cases, they still convey the pervasive idea that only certain types of women are deemed appropriate mothers. In other words, it is not enough to *be* a mother, but, to be socially accepted, a woman must be a *good* mother. The definition of good motherhood is based on notions of what makes a bad mother, much of which is rooted in ideas about class and race (Cooey 1999; Earle and Letherby 2003). Mainstream ideas about womanhood, motherhood, and family depict the heterosexual, white, middle-class, married woman as the most highly valued mother. All other women—including single mothers, poor mothers, mothers of color, and lesbian mothers—fall outside this narrow definition of the good mother. Thus, the mothering of such groups is often criticized and devalued (Arendell 2000; McCormack 2005).

Because the groups considered bad mothers are many times portrayed as social problems, their mothering practices are scrutinized more thoroughly, which perpetuates the bad mother label (McMahon 1995). Social agencies such as welfare departments and child protective services publicly survey the parental behavior of poor and working-class women. This surveillance amplifies the deviance of poor women by making their mothering practices far more visible than the mothering of higher-class groups (Blum 1999). Additionally, as relayed in this chapter's introduction, the mass media both reflect and perpetuate cultural stereotypes of bad mothers. Decades of media descriptions of the underclass blame poor women for perpetuating a "cycle of poverty" in which myriad social problems—from delinquency to failure in school—are linked exclusively to the home. In this sense, poor women are constructed as breeders of the underclass (Abramovitz 1995).

Although portrayed as *social* problems, many times the social reasons behind mothering practices go unnoticed by focusing on the individual characteristics of improper mothers rather than the social forces at play in their lives. Instead of addressing the poverty and the educational and employment disadvantages faced routinely by poor and working-class women, the media, policymakers, and others represent bad motherhood as the failure of individual women to carry out their maternal responsibilities properly. The different social contexts in which women live are disregarded, as are the differences in mothering that may ensue.

As I argue in this chapter, the binary distinction of good and bad motherhood that permeates stereotypes of mothering oversimplifies the experience. In the following pages I begin to examine the nuances in the categories of good mothers and bad mothers and demonstrate the ambiguity of such labels. For example, both women of low and high SES define good mothers as "being there" for their children. But, being there for women of high SES is reflective of the intensive mothering ideology and involves much more active participation in a child's life. Ultimately, I explore how women adapt to the larger social and cultural forces at play: how do women of low SES respond to mothering marginality, and how do women of high SES respond to mothering centrality? Studying these questions among infertile women is ideal because they are purposefully trying to enter a role for which they are viewed as either worthy or unworthy of attaining.

What Makes a Mother "Good"?

As family scholars Lawrence Ganong and Marilyn Coleman (1995, 511) suggest, "Despite the pressure on women to bear children due to the idealization of motherhood, just being a mother is not enough; being an appropriate type of mother is crucial." The women's desires to mother go beyond the motherhood mandate. Not only do all the women in this study want to mother, but they also all want to mother *well*. Despite the "myth" of good motherhood (Berry 1993; Thurer 1994), all study participants believed they are (or will be) good mothers. What I term the "good mother syndrome" permeated the women's discussions about motherhood, regardless of their social location. According to Barbara, an unemployed black woman of low SES, the belief that she is a good mother is her reason for wanting children: "I have always liked babies, you know, and I thought I would be good at it. You know, I thought I had something to actually share with a—a little person and, and just wanted it."

Deborah, a thirty-nine-year-old white woman of low SES, also describes her belief that she would be a good mother by relaying others' opinions about her potential: "In fact, everybody always told me, 'I'm the one person who should have kids.' I mean if they're looking around because, you know, I was always good with kids." Similarly, Nadia and Iris, white women of high SES, also believe they will be good mothers. Nadia told me, "I think I would be—I think I would be a very good mother." And, Iris explains, "I think that I'm good [at mothering]. Not great at it or anything but good at it. And so part of me I think is just—wants it innately and part of me thinks that it's—I'm good at the job."

But how do the women define what it means to be a good mother? Examining their definitions provides an initial glimpse into how the women begin to justify desiring such a role. Edin and Kefalas (2005, 10) first described poor women's definition of good mothering as "summed up in two words—being there." They suggest that this definition of good parenting is unique to the lower classes; however, this two-word phrase was the universal definition for good motherhood among all the women in this study, both poor and rich, black and white. Upon closer examination, however, what it means to "be there" varies among the classes and depends upon the women's social circumstances. Women adapt their definitions of good mothering to what they are able to provide. For women of low SES, this includes being present in the child's life, but for women of high SES "being there" is much more intense, indicative of the intensive mothering ideology that requires mothering to be "child-centered, expert-guided, emotionally absorbing, labor-intensive, and financially expensive" (Hays 1996, 8). The women mold their definitions of good motherhood to claim the status.

Veronica, a single black woman of low SES, exemplifies the responses given by the participants of low SES as to what makes a good mother: "Well, they have to be able to look out for their child. Help with the schoolwork. Don't lay around. Play with 'em. Just be there for 'em." Lynn, a white woman of low SES experiencing secondary infertility because she is currently unable to become pregnant but has a child from a previous pregnancy, similarly states: "I think good moms are ones that show up. And I think good moms are the ones that are able to protect their kids from bad things happening. And I think good moms are there."

For women of low SES, "being there" is composed of necessities and capabilities present in their own circumstances, such as "showing up" and "protecting" children from "bad things." The women also define good motherhood according to what *not* to do, such as "laying around," which they view as a predominant trait of mothering in their surroundings. Their concerns do not encompass idealized notions of good mothering such as the amount of interaction in a child's life and the intensity of that action. Such characteristics, however, are apparent in the responses of women of high SES, as Sarah, a mild-mannered speech therapist, suggests: "[A good mother is] somebody who's there and shares almost everything with you. Probably almost too much. My goodness. [My mother and I] did everything together and so it was like we shopped, we cooked, we cleaned. We—she would pick out my clothes. She would help me get dressed. She would take me to church. She would take me to Sunday school. She would do my homework with me. Ooh, boy (cries)." Courtney echoes Sarah's sentiments:

> A good mother is somebody who loves their children unconditionally and who will I mean basically lay down their life for their children. I'm not saying you have to give up your life and give up everything you are. Obviously moms are entitled to have a life and that's why I have my seven best friends. But, you know, someone who is selfless and giving to their children makes a good mother. And there's certain moms who are not able to run and play catch and, you know, you know, people with disabilities or people who aren't physically fit and active. And it doesn't mean they can't be a good mom. There's ways around everything. It's just having that desire to—to be active and—and—and interactive in your child's life.

The complexity of these descriptions, particularly the *active* engagement in a child's life cast in a language of self-sacrifice and unconditional love, distinguishes high SES women's definitions of good motherhood from those of women of low SES. Such *conceptual* differences parallel sociologist Annette Lareau's (2003) findings on social-class differences in mothering *practices*. She found that middle-class women undertake "concerted cultivation" of their children's talents by closely supervising their education and organizing after-school activities. This more active role in child rearing contrasts with poor and working-class mothers' parenting practices that Lareau calls "the accomplishment of natural growth," in which children are allowed more leniency in their free time.

The classed definitions of "being there" allowed the women to have different ideas about when they were ready to be (good) mothers. Because all participants were intentionally trying to mother at some point, all believed they were ready to undertake the role. For women of low SES, readiness to mother meant finding a job and housing. Women of high SES, by contrast, were ready to mother as determined by the typical path of life stages (for example, school, career, marriage, children), as well as by financial stability. That is, women of low SES reshaped mainstream notions of when women are ready to mother based on their own circumstances while women of high SES were bound to those notions.

The idea that people should not have a child unless they can afford one has permeated mainstream discussions of parenting (Solinger 2013). In the early twentieth century, the psychologist John Watson argued that "no one should have a child until she could afford to give the child a room of its own" (Ehrenreich and English 1979). Although this idea is present in professional and popular discussions of motherhood, poor and working-class women do not adhere to such prescriptions. Instead, they focus on things they *are* able to provide and achieve within the limits of their economic circumstances. Rachelle, a black woman of low SES in her late twenties, focuses on her mental state when determining her readiness to have a child:

> Well, a lot of people—I think a lot of people like put [readiness] on finances. I mean finances is a big, huge part of it but I think more like just your mind state because you could have like all the money in the world but if you're not mentally ready, you won't be able to take care of them still. Like some people get, you know, depressed and stuff like that and they have money and you still can't take care of 'em. You might have to hire somebody to help you: nannies or take 'em to family members' and stuff. So I think like if your mind isn't ready, it's no good.

Rachelle recognizes the dominant view that readiness depends upon finances. Yet, she rejects this idea by claiming that psychological readiness trumps finances in determining readiness to mother. Rachelle's shift in emphasis allows her to believe that she is ready to "be there" for a child, despite her economic circumstances.

Economics, however, was of utmost importance to women of high SES in determining when they should have a child. Sarah asks, "Are we ready for this? Can we really afford this?" Her queries demonstrate how higher-class women conflate affordability with readiness when making childbearing decisions. Nan's experience in determining when to have a child further illustrates this point:

> And then we got to a point where—where I guess both of us but more so me became more anxious to start trying, you know, kind of ready, you know,

to—to try. And really the only thing that was holding us back at that point was—was the income decision, you know, it got to a point where do I continue to work, have a baby, do the childcare thing or try to do it part—try to work part-time or—and then what ended up happening is Rick got offered a full salaried position at the university which provided us an income so that I could leave Ford to be at home full-time. So that's the point in time that we were overjoyed or happy. We were excited and in a position to be able to try to conceive. So.

For Rick and Nan, their readiness to have a child was contingent on the "income decision." Such a decision, however, encompassed far more than just income or money. Nan ideally wanted to quit her job so that she could stay at home with the child. Thus, embedded within their timing of childbearing was not only the norm of financial stability but also the norm of being a stay-at-home mom. Nan's decision to have a child was based on both the economic security of a middle-class lifestyle and her ability to adhere to a traditional gender ideology in which good mothers stay at home with their children.

For women of low SES, the primary indicator of readiness to parent was the exact opposite of higher-class benchmarks: women of low SES sought to get a job rather than the opportunity to quit a job. Overwhelmingly, the women of low SES mentioned having secure housing and/or a steady job as measures of being ready to mother. For these women, economic concerns centered on a more attainable goal: they sought a steady job, even if that job did not pay well, rather than a fluctuating, unstable source of income. Jewel, a white woman of low SES with several piercings and tattoos, reflects on the economics of motherhood: "I think if you have a job and you can take care of yourself then you should be able to take care of another child. If you don't have a job, you're living at home and everybody else is paying for you, it's not their burden to pay for your child, too. And I don't think you should have it in your mind, 'Oh, well, the state will pay for this and the state will pay for that.' I don't believe that either." Reflecting on the experiences of other mothers in her community, Jewel believes that having a job makes women ready to mother because it gives them independence—independence from both their families and the state. Jewel adopts the dominant view that condemns welfare dependency, yet she also makes motherhood attainable for herself by linking stability to occupation rather than to income.

Similarly, Keisha, a petite black woman of low SES in her early thirties, determines her readiness to mother by adapting her contextual norms to dominant ideals: "So (pauses) I wanted to at least be grown. I didn't want to be like a lot of young girls is having kids so I didn't want to be like that. And I wanted to be a little bit stable at least a place to stay and, you know, things like that: a job and things like that. So when I—really when I hit eighteen." Given a social context in which teenagers are frequently having children, stability to Keisha is having a place to stay and a job. Her immediate circumstances dictate norms that differ from the mainstream, including being "grown" at eighteen years of age and thus ready to mother. In other words, stability and the criteria for readiness to mother are relative to one's immediate circumstances.

While women of both high and low SES discussed, albeit differently, money and jobs as prerequisites to parenting, certain topics only arose in particular economic groups. Decreased partying is one such characteristic, mentioned exclusively by women of low SES. Echoing the "motive of redemptive mothering" in their reasons for wanting to mother, poor and working-class women believe they are ready to mother when they are no longer interested in the party lifestyle because motherhood will provide them with adult characteristics (McMahon 1995). Tanya, a married, white woman of low SES, observes:

> I don't know if I just grew up or—or what . . . When I was a teenager or early twenties and then finally it was like, "Well, I guess it's time to buckle down and do what you're going to do instead of just having fun." . . . I can't think of anything that really had happened. Maybe just hearing that from my friends growing—growing up and doing the same—not the same thing but—but finally had a—a way to go, you know, in life instead of just partying or shopping or hanging out or whatever. I think that was it . . . I already had a good job. I had a good job so I knew about responsibility and that part was no problem.

Tanya's peers revealed to her that having children gave meaning to their lives, something she was ready to attain. As she grew older, she felt that it was time to "buckle down," and having children allowed her to do that. Tanya also reiterates the importance of having a job when deciding to have children. Working gave her responsibility, a necessary characteristic for mothering.

As Rachelle previously mentioned in her rejection of the importance of money to being a good mother, many women of low SES believe having a stable mental state is of utmost importance when having a child. Keisha, a black woman of low SES, elaborates: "A stable life period. Basically it's a stable life. Even if you not with somebody and you— . . . you've just got to have a good life: a good mind, you know, you've got to have a good heart. You've got to—because kids just not something you just have. You know, you—they there, you've got to teach 'em so they can grow and be, you know, so yeah. You've got to have a good mind, a house, a home and life (laughs)." Keisha recognizes the fragility and responsibility that come with parenting. Thus, a "good mind" is necessary to teach children. Keisha is ready to mother because she has a "stable life" that encompasses a good "mentality" and a house.

Women of high SES did not mention emotional stability or partying when characterizing readiness to mother. Instead, reflecting their mothering motivations, they repeatedly mentioned sequential life stages as dictating their fertility timing. Courtney describes the benchmarks of readiness to parent: "I had planned on having children more towards my mid-twenties but my husband and I weren't in a hurry to get married. You know, we were both in school and we both wanted to be out of school and pretty well settled and have good careers under our belts before we moved forward with that." Courtney was not ready to have children until she reached that stage in her life. School, marriage, career, and then children are typical steps in the middle- and upper-class life-course trajectory. Adhering to mainstream ideas, the women knew they were ready to mother once certain milestones were achieved. Encompassed in this trajectory were life goals that went beyond motherhood, but women of low SES did not foresee such opportunities; for many of them motherhood was their ultimate goal. Brooke, a tall white woman of high SES, relays the typical sequence for many middle- and upper-class women; they were ready to mother once other goals were accomplished.

> I mean I knew I had other goals for myself besides just [having children] and I knew I was going to go to college. I knew even going to get my bachelor's degree I was going to go back and get a graduate degree. And so I had that goal that I—I was going to be educated and successful but I knew that once I had completed that or was close to completing that that I knew that I wanted to have children. And I knew that was going to be an important part of my life and that that—that being educated and successful was only going to be a part of who I was but the most important thing was having a family like I had when I was growing up.

Brooke had personal goals for herself beyond motherhood. She wanted to attain an education prior to having children. Additionally, Brooke adopted the intensive mothering ideology in her belief that she was to make family the center of her life as it was to be "the most important thing in her life." Unlike women of low SES who repeatedly described circumstances in their lives they did not want to mirror, women of high SES wanted to emulate their own childhood environment, such as Brooke's desire to have "a family like I had when I was growing up."

Not Just "Good," but Better: The Practice of Comparative Mothering

In addition to utilizing the resources at hand to prove their mothering capabilities, the participants did "comparative mothering" in which they compared their (hypothetical) mothering practices to others. Although all women practiced comparative mothering, how and why they did so differed by social class. Both socioeconomic groups compared themselves to bad mothers, but who those bad mothers comprised (for example, family and friends or strangers at the mall) differed among the women of high and low SES. Additionally, unlike women of high SES, women of low SES compared themselves to poorer women, an effort to distance themselves from that demographic group, and they used comparative mothering to redefine what it means to be a good mother.

Sociologists David Snow and Leon Anderson (1987) first studied how marginalized individuals (for example, homeless people) form identities that do not reflect the stigmatized stereotypes associated with their social group. The question of how individuals construct their own sense of meaning and value in a context that gives them none is one that can be applied to the women of low SES and their pursuit of motherhood in this study. The participants practice what Snow and Anderson call "distancing identity work." Such work typically occurs when there is an incongruity between an individual's self-concept (for example, *I* am a good mother) and her role-based, social identity (for example, poor women are bad mothers). Rather than simply accepting this social identity, the women actively construct and negotiate personal identities that are consistent with their self-concepts. They often do so through comparative mothering, in which they distance themselves from poor women who are bad parents.

Women of low SES first compare themselves to their own mothers in an effort to move away from the bad mother stereotype. Regina, a married, black woman of low SES, explains: "I'll make sure that I [don't] treat my kids the way I was treated. You know. And I wanted—I [don't] want them to grow up the way I grew up."

Jewel, a white woman of low SES, further reveals that she can be a good mother because her own deprived upbringing has taught her what *not* to do: "I think I'd be a good mother for what I've dealt with through my childhood. I know how you're not supposed to treat your kids, I know how you're supposed to treat your kids and I just—I would like to be a mother. I would—I feel very strongly that I could be a good mother and take care of my child." According to Jewel, she knows how "you're not supposed to treat your kids" due to her own treatment as a child. Her own biography gives her confidence in her mothering abilities and allows her to overcome the construction of poor women as unfit mothers.

Beyond their familial situations, women of low SES also distance themselves from bad mothers in their current circumstances. Doing so is one way women of low SES justify their desire of a role for which they are portrayed as unsuitable. Angie, a black woman of low SES, dissociates herself from the stereotype of bad mother by describing other women in these terms: ". . . And there's some people out there who don't want kids and leave their kids on the porch at below-zero weather and beat their kids and abuse their kids. Like I hate watching the news. Some of the stuff just kills me. Like God knows I'll probably be the best mother. Why is somebody that would treat their kid like that deserve to have a kid and I can't?" Comparing themselves to these more extreme, well-publicized images allows the women of low SES to detach from their own contexts and thus justify their desire for children. Doing so was commonplace among this group as Lisa, a white woman of low SES, refers to the "Octomom" as the epitome of inappropriate mothering—someone "who takes advantage of things like [welfare]."

In addition to comparing themselves to sensationalized constructions of bad mothers, the poor and working-class women in this study identified bad mothers in their own communities, typically among individuals close to them. Jewel, a white woman of low SES, describes the deterioration of a friendship, given her impatience with her friend's poor mothering:

> One of my friends I'm not really friends with anymore. She had a child when she was seventeen and that child lives with her grandmother. She doesn't see that child, doesn't come over and spend the night or anything. Like she's in this life but she doesn't take care of it. And she went out and she has—she's pregnant again and she's going to be due in July and this baby's going to be living with her but her other child's going to be living with her grandmother. And I don't look highly on people that are like that. . . . That's why we're not friends. So . . . I just—I know that I would be such a good mother and for her to be able to have a kid, I resent her for her to be able to do that when she's not going to take care of it. And that's like everybody.

Jewel does not approve of her friend's familial situation and current pregnancy. Through her disapproval she is able to distance herself from that type of mothering and construct herself as "such a good mother." It is interesting that the women of low SES utilize *both* mainstream depictions of bad mothering, as in the case of Angie watching the news, as well as mothering in their own communities, such as that described by Jewel; this combination demonstrates the heterogeneity, or mixture of ideas, present in the poor and working-class environments (Harding 2007). Both ideology and context converge to shape their experiences.

Women of high SES also engage in comparative mothering, but they do so for different reasons. Rather than criticize and distance themselves from their families of origin, middle- and upper-class women wanted to emulate their mothers' actions. Stephanie, a substitute teacher, describes her own background: "We—so [my parents] were very family conscious and I—I could see us doing that as well and longed for those interactions. So I could see that in my future and replicating some of that and the memories, you know, traditions." Stephanie wants to "replicate" her childhood memories through her own role as a mother. As part of the dominant class, Stephanie is able to maintain her past experiences and not sacrifice the good mother characterization in doing so. Women of low SES, in contrast, must distance themselves from their bad childhoods in order to claim good motherhood for themselves.

Like the women of low SES in this study, however, women of high SES did distance themselves from those considered to be bad mothers according to social ideals. Carole describes a bad mother she encountered: "That scumball has six of 'em. Look, she's not even watching and that one's in the faucet and that one is in the fountain, you know, of the mall. I could take you, you, you, you and nobody would even notice. Not that you would obviously. I'm not saying I'm a kidnapper but you wonder how some of these, you know—some of these kids, you think, 'Geez, I'd be doing you a favor (laughs).' Some of these ladies would probably say, 'Yeah, go ahead. Take it (laughs). I didn't want her anyway.' So (pauses)." In describing the mothering of women she observes in the mall whose children she should "kidnap" to improve their lives, Carole implies that her mothering skills are superior. Additionally, through her description, Carole employs many stereotypical characterizations of bad mothers, such as their young age, implicit in her use of "kids" and the belief that bad mothers unintentionally have children since they "don't want them anyway."

Nadia also makes similar comparisons: "I think I would be—I think I would be a very good mother. . . . I could be a better mom with my hands tied behind my back and my eyes closed than some of these idiots I see raising kids. You know, you just walk through the—the grocery store and the way the—the interactions you see between parents and children is just appalling. . . . Nobody is perfect. But I think I'd do a hell of a job and I think I'd do—be a really good mom."

When doing comparative mothering, participants of high SES tended to criticize women they observed in public places, such as the mall or grocery store. Such ethnically and socioeconomically diverse venues allow middle- and upper-class women to interact with people outside of their typical social settings. Women of high SES are already distanced from the sensationalized news stories that Angie alluded to, and they do not have the intimate exposure to family and friends stereotyped as bad mothers so they utilize behavior in public places as a mechanism to maintain themselves as "better" mothers. Additionally, unlike women of low SES, the participants of high SES used derogatory epithets to further characterize bad mothers, such as Carole's use of "scumball" and Nadia's reference to "idiots." Perhaps they do so because of the class distance that exists between them and those they characterize—a distance that allows them to belittle the "other." By contrast, women of low SES do not have the luxury of such a distance from those whom they are criticizing.

While women of both high and low SES used comparative mothering to distance themselves from worse mothers, only poor and working-class women used comparative mothering to distance themselves from an impoverished identity. They needed this additional distancing because of a social identity that conflates class status with mothering ability. Roxanne, a single, black woman of low SES, attempts to distance herself from the label of being poor by comparing her situation to women in more dire straits: "My god-sister calls me like, 'I'm seven months pregnant.' . . . She's like—but I'm like, 'You're eighteen and you have two kids now. And you're like not financially stable.' I mean at least I am in a place where I can like take care of a baby if I was to have one." By criticizing her god-sister for "not being financially stable" yet becoming pregnant, Roxanne distinguishes herself from poor women even though her annual income is less than $10,000—a number that is far below all recent determinations of the federal poverty level. In distancing herself from poverty, Roxanne rejects her exclusion from motherhood, but, in doing so, she further reinforces the notion that poor women are not good mothers.

In addition to using comparative mothering to distance themselves from negative stereotypes, the women of low SES uniquely used that practice to expand the notion of what it means to be a good mother. Women of high SES, however, did not use comparison in that manner because ideas of good mothering already apply to them. These findings similarly reflect Pierrette Hondagneu-Sotelo and Ernestine Avila's research (1997) in which they found that transnational Latina nannies applied the ideals of intensive mothering to their employers who had significant material resources. The nannies developed more flexible notions of good motherhood for themselves given their limited finances as well as their physical separation from their children. In other words, the nannies conceived of themselves as good mothers by manipulating the ideology of motherhood and tailoring it to their situations.

Similarly, in this study, Carrie, a white woman of low SES previously employed as a nanny, explains that in her community, time spent with children is what makes a good mother. She expands the definition of good mothering by noting that wealthy women who are typically recognized as good mothers may not live up to that ideal. In this sense, Carrie rejects the stereotypical notion that places class at the center of good mothering.

> And I know I'm sure people think, "If you can't afford to have kids, then you can't afford to have kids (laughs). If you can't afford to make the kids, then you can't afford to have kids." I mean it's true. I really can't afford to have children. I can't. Does that mean that I shouldn't? My neighbors next door are doing it. I can do it better than them. . . . I mean really it's not a problem with me. It's a problem with the society that the gap between the rich and poor is so big and I mean I'd like to think that if I could afford a Hummer, I wouldn't drive one. You know, I'd like to think I am more s—conscious than those people. So just because they have money, it's not making them better or better parents. . . . I would rather live in a trailer and spend time with my children than live in a mansion and—and have to work all of those hours to live in that mansion (laughs).

Carrie acknowledges her exclusion from good motherhood according to her social class, but, when comparing her projected parenting style to that of her employers, Carrie dismisses the current ideals around mothering because she recognizes that wealth and good motherhood do not necessarily go hand in hand. In turn, she redefines what it means to be a good mother given her own circumstances and what she can provide. Carrie can "do it better" by reconceptualizing the idea of good motherhood, in which time spent with children takes precedence over material resources.

Jodi, a short, single white woman of low SES, also rejects the dominant notion of good motherhood and redefines it according to her situation.

> ANN: And have you asked [the doctors] specifically about getting pregnant?
> JODI: Mm-hm.
> ANN: And what has their response been?
> JODI: "Are you really ready? Are you sure you want one? It's a lot of work." "I wouldn't be asking if I didn't know that" (laughs). . . . I mean I know it's [the doctors'] job so and they just want to, you know, be cautious because there are so many people that end up having, you know, that's what I don't get. It's like you have people that really want children, you know . . . really want them when the time is right. And then you have kids that have kids or other people that have them and just either do horrible things to them or,

you know, just it's—they know they should—they should not have a child
(laughs). And they're not ready.

Given her young age, marital status, and low income, physicians have questioned Jodi's readiness to have children. In reflecting upon these encounters, Jodi compares herself to others to reveal how even individuals who
conform to the dominant understanding of good mothers, and thus are
expected to be ready to have children, might not always be good parents.
Jodi expands the concept of good mothering to emphasize the desire for
children. To her, readiness to have children is not based on demographic
characteristics; rather, readiness is based on the longing and desire for
parenting.

Ebony, a black woman of low SES in her mid-thirties, sums it up well
when she states: "Because even people—and it's kind of weird because even
people with money maybe don't treat their kids the same as people who
don't have money. . . . Because just because you have money don't mean
you're going to treat people right or just because you necessarily don't have
as much money, you might treat people better because you know how it
feels to not be as fortunate. So yeah." Ebony does not equate being a good
parent with having money. In fact, she turns her misfortune into an advantage and a reason to assert that she is actually a good mother.

The participants use the practice of comparative mothering in two strategic ways. First, women of both high and low SES distance themselves
from negative stereotypes of bad mothers by categorizing other women
in those terms. This identity work reinforces the binary of fit versus unfit
mothers. The women accept the ideology, but they reject the idea that it
applies to them, thereby reinforcing the very forces that they are trying to
overcome (Nelson 2002). While accepting the good/bad mother binary,
women of low SES additionally use comparative mothering to challenge
the *content* of that binary. They redefine what it means to be a good mother
by exposing the inadequacy of dominant conceptions of good motherhood. At the same time, they point to features of their own lives that allow
them to attain the good motherhood ideal. In this way, both groups of
women use the same technique, comparison, to actively resist the label of
bad mother. The women construct their own hierarchies of motherhood,
according to which other women, whether richer or poorer than themselves, are more inadequate mothers than they are (Collins 1990).

In a literature review on motherhood, sociologist Terry Arendell (2000) identified four main gaps in research on motherhood that deserve further study: identities and meanings of motherhood; relational aspects; experiences of mothering; and contextual settings from within which women mother. Arendell recognized the lack of understanding of marginalized motherhood and posed an unanswered question: "How do women actively resist the dominant ideologies of mothering and family?" The findings in this chapter begin to answer this question. Understanding how and why women purposefully pursue a status from which they are excluded or viewed as unfit reveals how they rework definitions of good mothering to fit the circumstances of their lives.

Regardless of their race or class, all the women grappled with their social circumstances and ideological notions to construct themselves as good mothers. The "good mother syndrome" was achieved through adaptive definitions of what makes a good mother, demonstrated through both women's readiness to mother and the mechanism of comparative mothering. The women of high and low SES differed along all those lines, and by examining those differences this chapter exposes the importance of class to motherhood: from shaping how motherhood is defined (and the intensity of "being there") to determining to whom women compare themselves (family members or strangers). Beyond these negotiations with ideologies of good motherhood, the women actively attempt to pursue their desire to mother.

3

"Getting Pregnant's a Piece of Cake"

• •

Trying to Mother

[Pregnancy] maybe happens in between or it maybe happens whenever it just decides to pop up. But I don't really think when you plan it—it helps.
—Roxanne, black woman of low SES

You know, we did sort of the normal stuff. . . . Well, I did a little reading. I got, you know, a couple of books. And, you know, we'd go to Borders . . . and I'd sit there with a stack of fertility books. And, you know, I tried a few dietary things, although I've never been great at that. And then we did, you know, started doing the temperature . . . and so that's what we did at first.
—Colleen, white woman of high SES

Throughout the course of my interviews, as I asked the women to describe their process of trying to become pregnant, I realized that the way researchers currently frame pregnancy intentions (along race and class lines) is deeply flawed. In defining intent in terms of "conscious action," such as planning, deciding, or trying to conceive, national surveys and researchers exclude the pregnancy intentions of economically marginalized women. For women of low SES whose lives do not allow for a prioritization of such active planning, constructing childbearing intent in such a manner fails to capture their purposeful pursuits and desires for pregnancy.

Few studies have explored pregnancy intentions among women of low SES, but those few have found that the concept "planned a pregnancy" is not meaningful to many low-income women. Women of low SES rarely admit to making a conscious decision to have children (Moos et al. 1997). Instead, unacknowledged decisions or nondecisions inform their childbearing pursuits, which in turn become categorized as *un*intentional. In other words, conflating intent with trying, planning, or deciding as many researchers currently do (for example, Greil and McQuillan 2010; Mayer 1997), labels low SES women's pregnancies falsely and negatively as "unintended." As a result, the significantly higher rate of unintended pregnancies among poor women reported by the National Survey of Family Growth may be a product of miscategorization, owing to class-specific conceptualization. My research, however, on women who viewed themselves as *involuntarily* childless and thus all intending to become pregnant, reveals how women of low SES do indeed intend to become pregnant but *conceive* of such intent differently from the women of high SES; thus, they would not be captured in current measurements of childbearing intent.

Such faulty categorization negatively affects poor and working-class women. Planned pregnancies and control over one's fertility are valued in American society, while unintentional pregnancies are viewed as problematic (Barrett and Wellings 2002; Greil and McQuillan 2010; Luker 1996; Nathanson 1991). Restricting childbearing intent to planning, deciding, or trying to become pregnant excludes the experiences of economically marginalized women, despite their active desire for children. This conceptualization further stigmatizes women of low SES as deviant, while women of high SES, whose practices follow the normative scripts of intent, are seen more positively. In other words, the way we socially construct the "social problem" of unintended pregnancies maintains the stratified system of reproduction in the United States (Colen 1986; Ginsburg and Rapp 1991). Poor and working-class women are stereotyped as reproductively negligent and unfit mothers, while middle- and upper-class white women are deemed maternally competent and good mothers.

Past researchers have echoed these concerns by highlighting the classist basis of the measurement of intent and its failure to capture poor and working-class women's experiences (Augustine, Nelson, and Edin 2009; Moos et al. 1997). Studies have also recently explored the concept of ambivalence within intention as well, such as the idea that women are "okay either way" (McQuillan, Greil, and Shreffler 2011). But for women who view pregnancy more fatalistically as something that just happens, the concept of ambivalence is inappropriate because it reflects not their ambivalence about becoming pregnant per se, but rather a lack of concern about the timing and number of pregnancies (Klerman 2000). *Why,* I wondered, does the meaning of intent differ among women of various social classes, and *why* is planning not meaningful to women of low SES, in particular? Exploring such questions not only provides a deeper understanding of intent, but it also elaborates upon the dynamics, practices, and ideologies at play in reproduction and childbearing more generally.

Trying to Mother

Despite the recent increase in media attention to infertility and reproductive technologies, infertility remains a relatively silent issue, particularly in relation to its antithesis, pregnancy. Therefore, most women in the study, regardless of race or class, believed that pregnancy would be an "easy thing" to achieve and had high expectations for success before starting on their journeys. Carrie, a white woman of low SES, "just thought it would be easy and didn't think anything of it," and Jennifer, a white woman of high SES, believed that "getting pregnant's going to be no big deal . . . that's, you know, a piece of cake."

Based on this premise of ease and with their desire for children intact, the women engaged in a variety of processes to become pregnant. These processes differed by social class, primarily around the planning components of intent. Women of low SES who want to conceive do not try to become pregnant in the sense that they do not deliberately decide when or how they will achieve conception; rather, their actions—not using contraception—imply their desire for as well as their purposeful pursuit of pregnancy. By contrast, women of high SES deliberately decide to become pregnant and employ specific technological mechanisms to achieve pregnancy in a certain time frame.

Such differences reflect both structural and cultural variations between the social classes. Structurally, women of low SES have less access to knowledge and resources pertaining to reproduction than do women of high SES. And culturally, there are differences in the importance of control over reproduction among women of different social classes (Lazarus 1994; Zadoroznyj 1999). The idea that motherhood should be planned reflects higher-class women's circumstances, yet it ignores the lack of perceived control over sexuality present in the restricted contexts of poor and working-class women's lives (Hill 2004).

Women of low SES did not decide when, where, or how to become pregnant. Instead, as Roxanne puts it, they waited for the pregnancy to "pop up": "Because it's like I know a lot of people that it's like, 'Okay, well, I'm going to get this job and then I'm going to do this and I'm going to buy this car and then I'm going to try to work on the baby.' And it doesn't happen that way. It maybe happens in between or it maybe happens whenever it just decides to pop up. But I don't really think when you plan it— it helps." Roxanne is aware of the typical life-course trajectory in which women of high SES believe. In her experiential context, however, life just "doesn't happen that way"; therefore, she does not see planning as helpful to achieving pregnancy. Roxanne does not undertake the conscious action of deciding when or how to achieve pregnancy; rather, the pregnancy itself becomes the active player that "decides to pop up."

Because women of low SES do not believe it is possible to control the exact timing of pregnancy, they do not deliberately decide to try to become pregnant. As Judy, an unemployed white woman of low SES, demonstrates, an explicit conversation outlining childbearing intentions is not part of her discourse:

ANN: So did—was this a mutual decision? Did [your partner] want children as well?

JUDY: Mm-hm.

ANN: Tell me a little bit about that conversation when you talked about it.

JUDY: Well, I mean we didn't talk about it beforehand so much, but we didn't
   try to prevent it.

ANN: Okay.

JUDY: But he had—he wanted kids and so did I. He didn't have any kids, so.

Judy's quote demonstrates how intent is not equated with planning or decision making. She and her partner nevertheless fully intended to become pregnant; however, only her reference to wanting children hints at such a purpose. My questions, informed by my social position and the literature on infertility, were phrased using terms such as "decision" and "conversation," which did not speak to Judy's experience. She successfully reframed my ideas to fit her own circumstances, as she and her partner "didn't try," but the fact that they "wanted kids" implied intent and mutual decision making.

In fact, women of low SES literally rejected planning because they felt it interfered with nature. Carla, a married black woman of low SES, demonstrates this mindset in her response to my question if she did anything in particular to become pregnant besides not using contraception: "No . . . I like, you know, didn't try anything extraordinary. I didn't—nothing . . . I didn't time the day. I didn't know . . . Because I always felt like, 'Okay, if it's going to happen, it's just going to happen naturally, you know' . . . I don't want to have to—I don't want to have to plan it. It's like, no, I want the—I want to have the feeling at least to—to know it just—it was natural."

To Carla and most other participants of low SES planning a pregnancy was unnatural. Such reasoning may be a product of their contextual circumstances in which limited resources and knowledge about technological mechanisms to assist in achieving pregnancy (for example, temperature taking) restricted how they approached childbearing. Disadvantaged groups typically do not have the option of exercising choice and control around reproduction, making their reactions to childbirth appear more fatalistic (Zadoroznyj 1999).

Despite their apparent fatalism surrounding childbearing intent, women of low SES *did* consciously participate in acts to achieve pregnancy, primarily unprotected intercourse. In this sense, action coincides with intent, but they conceive and understand that action as natural and therefore do not view it as trying. Keisha, a black woman of low SES, exemplifies this reasoning:

ANN: What do you—do you do anything in particular with your current boyfriend to get pregnant?

KEISHA: No, we're just doing the regular way (laughs). . . . But we're not doing it really—not really (laughs)—I don't know—nothing crazy but (both laugh) just the regular way.

ANN: Having unprotected sex?

KEISHA: Yeah . . . That's—that's about it.

Keisha's statements demonstrate how the women of low SES in the study interpreted unprotected sex as natural or "regular," thereby depicting other mechanisms of achieving pregnancy as unnatural or "crazy." Tanya, a white woman of low SES, similarly believes "charting your temperature or your days or trying to keep up with when this was or when this was . . . is kind of like a clinical experiment or something." Additionally, the term "clinical" connotes inappropriate emotional detachment, which may cause the women of low SES to view the very process of taking their temperature as interfering with the spontaneity and emotional connection expected when having sex.

By equating unprotected sex with natural conception, these women of low SES may not acknowledge their actions as decisions, but they do recognize the consequences of such actions and undertake them with the intent of becoming pregnant, as Ebony, a vivacious black woman of low SES, demonstrates when she states: "Because if you're not using protection, you want kids. And that's my motto like, 'Okay, if you're not using protection, you do want kids.' It ain't—it wasn't a mistake. It's a mistake when you're young and you don't know and when you consciously know and you're an adult, you want kids flat out." Ebony's "motto" reveals the women's conscious understanding of the choice not to use contraception and the implications of doing so. The women of low SES actively choose not to use contraception with the intent of conceiving a child, but they do not acknowledge it as a decision or plan because they view it as a natural part of intending to become pregnant.

Barbara, a mild-mannered black woman of low SES, further displays how the women are conscious of the effects of not using contraception and purposefully avoid birth control in order to achieve pregnancy: "I am very up front about it that 'I'm not using any kind of birth control so, you know, this is what could happen. And if this does happen, this is what is going to happen as a result of it.' And so but I just assume by consent. But [my partners are] in by—by actions maybe that there is consent." Barbara hopes to become pregnant by having unprotected intercourse with several different partners. She is "up front" about her intentions to become pregnant and "assumes" that the act of not using contraception implies the partner's consent. This is clearly a deliberate plan to achieve pregnancy, yet Barbara does not conceive of it as such because unprotected sex is viewed as natural and associated with casualness and informality.

The white women of low SES also used unprotected sex as their mechanism to achieve pregnancy, yet, as the previous examples demonstrate, the black women of low SES were much more forthright in the level of consciousness associated with that decision. Perhaps that is because in the culture of black women of low SES the act of having sex itself is associated with a pursuit of pregnancy. Tamara, a black woman of low SES, told me, "Well, you know, most young girls the first time they have sex they almost about ready, you know, to get pregnant." Such thinking could be attributed to an "alternative life-course strategy" present in black, low-income communities in which younger childbearing is seen as more acceptable than in white communities, a distinction marked by differing sociocultural constraints, such as having limited opportunities beyond motherhood (Burton 1990; Furstenburg 1987). The increased acceptability of early, nonmarital parenthood in black communities may allow for an increased ease of conversation around having unprotected sex for the purpose of procreation in contrast to the low-income white women.

In addition to wanting a natural conception, many women of low SES rejected planning because it did not fit with their lifestyle. Ruby, a witty, married white woman of low SES, describes how regimented timing of intercourse does not mesh with the schedule of working-class couples:

ANN: What about like taking your temperature or—
RUBY: I have never tried it . . . never. . . . We did it so many times, I didn't think there was a moment we could have missed. At all. And if there wasn't a moment we missed, I don't think there would be any temperature time. When he goes to work, I can't call and say, "Come home from work."

Ruby works the day shift as an aide at a children's center while her husband works the night shift at a local factory. He is not home in the mornings when it is assumed to be the best time to take one's temperature and subsequently have intercourse if indicated that ovulation is occurring. In the current economic climate, many participants were in long-distance relationships because their partners worked in other states where they could find employment. This was the case for Judy, which meant for months at a time she was separated from her boyfriend, a lifestyle not conducive to planning a pregnancy. Such situations, intimately connected to economic circumstances, were not present in the lives of the women of high SES.

Finally, many women of low SES simply did not know how to try to become pregnant beyond unprotected intercourse. They were unfamiliar with mechanisms such as ovulation kits, temperature charts, or cervical mucus observations as fertility aides. Jocelyn, an introverted black woman of low SES, demonstrates:

> ANN: Did you take your temperature or, you know, [have intercourse] at a certain time of month or anything like that?
>
> JOCELYN: Oh, you're supposed to take your temperature? I didn't know you were supposed to take your temperature (both laugh). Really?

This lack of knowledge may be a result of less information sharing around reproduction in low-income settings. Black women of low SES, in particular, do not discuss personal issues as openly as their wealthier counterparts (Hill 2009). Additionally, more limited access to education and health care in disadvantaged settings hinders fertility knowledge.

Unlike women of low SES, the study participants of high SES explicitly planned, intended, and tried to become pregnant. Whereas the economically marginalized participants, such as Judy, did not have an overt conversation about attempting to become pregnant, women of high SES planned every detail in advance. Doing so reflects the typical life-course trajectory of women of high SES. They are ready to be mothers once they reach a certain life stage, usually after school, career, and marriage. Now that they have reached the childbearing stage, women of high SES attempt to be just as precise with their timing and planning. Sarah, a white woman of high SES, wanted to time her pregnancy so that it would not coincide with a holiday: "In the beginning it was like, 'I don't want to have a baby at Christmas so let's not work on it this month. Let's wait.'" Such statements are in stark contrast to the women of low SES who were hoping to have the pregnancy come on its own accord. Not only does Sarah want to schedule her pregnancy around certain events, but she also considers achieving pregnancy "work," which counters the low SES women's desires to become pregnant "naturally."

Women of high SES literally "take charge" of their fertility by researching how and when to become pregnant. Becca, a seemingly anxious white woman of high SES, states: "Well, you know, you take—I was taking my temperature . . . I read the book *Taking Charge of Your Fertility,* and so it tells you how to take your basal body temperature." Becca researched fertility planning prior to starting to try to become pregnant. She prepared for this next stage in her life so that she could successfully conceive; much like one would study for an exam in order to attain the desired grade. It gave her the sense that she was in control of how and when conception would occur, unlike women of low SES, such as Jocelyn, who did not know how temperature was related to fertility.

The messages and practices prevalent in communities become the norm for those living within that context. For women of low SES who intended to become pregnant, unprotected sex was the norm, whereas the norm for women of high SES included more technological mechanisms of trying. The differences reflect variation in the social and cultural context of pregnancy and demonstrate that the current definition of unintended pregnancies is inadequate because it is based on high SES conceptions of the "normal" practices associated with fertility intentions. Colleen, a tall, white woman of high SES, reflects on such middle- and upper-class ideas: "You know, we did sort of the normal stuff. . . . Well, I did a little reading. I got, you know, a couple of books. And, you know, we'd go to Borders . . . and I'd sit there with a stack of fertility books. And, you know, I tried a few dietary things, although I've never been great at that. And then we did, you know, started doing the temperature. . . . And so that's what we did at first. And I, you know, honestly didn't expect to get pregnant right away as much as I'd hoped that I would. I certainly thought I would within six months."

For Colleen and many other women of high SES in the study, the "normal stuff" of attempting to conceive included fertility research, diet alterations, temperature taking, and ovulation charting. In other words, there is a different sense of normal for the SES groups. Colleen's preparation for childbearing differs dramatically from the low SES women's desires to become pregnant naturally through the norm of unprotected intercourse. Such differences demonstrate that motherhood and reproduction are socially shaped by the intersection of race, class, and gender.

"We Ain't Got No Kid Yet": Recognizing Childbearing Difficulties

The intent to become pregnant is demonstrated by examining the participants' realizations of their childbearing difficulties. When women do not achieve their intended goal, pregnancy, they begin to realize that something is wrong. Because women differ in the mechanisms they use to achieve pregnancy, how, when, and why they recognize their childbearing difficulties vary between the classes. Given low SES women's less technical or strategic attempts at becoming pregnant, most did not think much about *not* becoming pregnant for quite some time. Erin, a white woman of low SES in her late thirties, is one example: "I mean it didn't actually occur to us that something might be wrong or different. . . . And I don't think it was our main focus. . . . We didn't miss a beat and we didn't try fertility, you know, we didn't try birth control of any sort so we just assumed it would happen eventually." Because of her belief that unprotected sex is natural and her fatalistic understanding that pregnancy would happen on its own accord, Erin "just assumed [pregnancy] would happen eventually." Because they are not adhering to fixed schedules, women of low SES allow more time to elapse before they recognize "that something might be wrong." "Two and a half years" go by before Barbara began wondering "what's going on here," while "three to four years" passed before Ebony started asking "why am I not getting pregnant?"

Having unprotected intercourse for such an extended period of time without conceiving was the first indication of childbearing difficulty for many participants of low SES. Donna, a cautious black woman of low SES, states: "And then it probably was like three years into it—three years into it it was like, 'Whoa. Wait a minute. We ain't got no kid yet.'" After avoiding contraception for three years without becoming pregnant, Donna realized that infertility might be a problem. Recognition of the issue implies that she was intending to become pregnant with unprotected intercourse, despite the lack of decision making or planning inherent within the dominant definition of intent.

In addition to having years of unprotected intercourse to no avail, women of low SES recognize their childbearing difficulties due to friends' and family members' pregnancies during the period they, themselves, tried unsuccessfully to become pregnant. Jodi, a white woman of low SES, explains:

ANN: When did you first realize that it was difficult for you to become pregnant?

JODI: Well, I had a theory all along because I didn't lose my virginity until two weeks after I turned eighteen. And then, you know, everybody—everybody around me: younger, older, my age, you know, every time I see 'em, they have a child or they have another child and another child. . . . But yeah, I—I mean there's obviously if you have unprotected sex and you're pregnant and like I never have. And I have—I have had unprotected sex. Yeah. You know, in my time and it just—it never happened.

Jodi assumed that after losing her virginity and having unprotected sex she would become pregnant. This was the norm in her community since "everyone around" her has children through those means. Jodi may not have planned for a pregnancy, per se, yet after having unprotected intercourse and "never" becoming pregnant she realizes her difficulties, thereby implicitly acknowledging her intentions. Such a contradiction among women of low SES demonstrates the importance of deciphering the nuance in conceptions of intent. The current definition of intent overlooks the experiences of women of low SES and fails to recognize their childbearing pursuits.

Unlike women of low SES who "do not think much about" becoming pregnant and recognize childbearing difficulties only after considerable time has elapsed, women of high SES realize their issues quickly and think about them actively. It took Brooke "three to four months" before she "first started kind of questioning" if there was a problem conceiving, while Becca waited "maybe five months" before becoming concerned.

While the women of low SES realize their fertility issues with the passage of time, a more passive acknowledgment, women of high SES take a more active role in understanding their difficulties through research. Sarah, a white woman of high SES, explains: "[I started researching on] the Internet. . . . Driving me up the wall. Yeah. Yeah, it was—yeah, it was really the Internet because I don't think I really knew anybody that— none of my friends have had this. So yeah, I think probably about six months. I was like, 'Yeah, you know,' and then it's my husband saying, 'Don't worry about it. It's normal. It could take a year. It could take over a year.' But yeah, then the worry sets in so. And you can't turn that off." After "about six months," Sarah began to "worry" that something was wrong. Because she did not know of any friends who had difficulties becoming pregnant and because of her husband's belief in the medical view that infertility should not be an issue until one year of trying, Sarah turned to the Internet for an explanation. She actively sought out information rather than waiting for time to pass.

Iris, an artistic white woman of high SES, similarly undertook research to understand her problems becoming pregnant: "And but then after six months it felt like it was not on—I don't know—I—I'm a winner and I like to succeed and I felt like the—the—our goal wasn't happening. . . . And I did way more research online. Like fanatical research online about when I could—we should have sex and—and other people who were having this and if I should be concerned yet and it didn't seem like I should and so." Iris was accustomed to being a "winner" and "succeeding" at things in life. The control and choice she usually was able to exercise were not inherent in her childbearing experience. Instead, actively engaging in research on the Internet helped her regain a sense of control in order to achieve her intended "goal" of pregnancy.

Given stereotypes of infertility, it is easy to assume that these differences may be age related. But, as acknowledged in the introduction, the differences I identified in my analyses fall to socioeconomic factors. Indeed, Brooke, Sarah and Iris are all under the age of thirty-five, and, after comparing responses by age, no differences were found; rather, the differences surfaced when comparing SES groups.

Unintended pregnancies, demonized in American popular culture and seen as indicative of irresponsible reproductive behavior, are thus used as a marker of a community's reproductive health. Policymakers, whether health educators or researchers, generalize about the phrase, without considering how women differ in their lived experiences, resources, and constraints. This chapter reveals the necessity of doing so because there are dramatic differences in the meaning of childbearing intentions among women in different social locations. Exposing such variation begins to ultimately reveal how mainstream understandings of intent are rooted in race- and class-based norms.

How women interpret fertility intent depends upon the context in which they live. Indeed, women of high SES subscribe to the stereotypical understandings of intent in which deciding and planning for childbearing are inherent in the very definition of the term. This conception reflects values present in the contexts of those with resources and power: choice and control. Choice and control, however, are taken-for-granted privileges of affluent women, not characteristic of more disadvantaged groups

(Dillaway and Brubaker 2006). Women of low SES, who have few choices and limited control over most life events, are more passive about becoming pregnant. Yet the intent to become pregnant, ever-present in their actions, is implicit in their act of unprotected sex and their disappointment when this strategy fails.

Class differences in the meaning of intent, then, reflect differences in the social context of women's lives. They are also shaped by broader cultural beliefs and ideologies relating to sex, pregnancy, and motherhood. For example, many teens do not use birth control because it would imply that they plan or intend to engage in sexual intercourse, which society deems amoral (Brubaker 2007). Similarly, for women of low SES and women of color, admitting to deliberately planning a pregnancy when they are ideologically portrayed as bad mothers is socially unacceptable. Therefore, by letting pregnancy happen on its own or at "God's will" allows marginalized women to compromise ideals of motherhood: they are able to satisfy the "motherhood mandate" by having children, yet not claim their purposeful pursuit of the negative stereotype of the unmarried, promiscuous, or otherwise bad mother. In other words, by not intentionally planning a baby, but passively accepting one if it should come along, women of low SES are able to assert a "modicum of respectability" (Augustine, Nelson, and Edin 2009, 113). Once women recognize their childbearing difficulties, they are confronted with having to live with them.

4

"Socioeconomically It Would Be Much More Difficult"

• •

The Lived Experience of Infertility

It's—I don't feel socially accepted some-times because all my friends now have children or are settling down and have children. None of them have problems, I guess. And I have quite a few friends. . . . But I don't feel socially accepted in any way. . . . We either are too young for the people or we don't have kids and we're not family. We're oddball. It just—I just—I just—a horrible thing.
—Ruby, white woman of low SES

So I think we've got a lot of support, which is nice. . . . You know, people that we can rely on not to judge and just be supportive and sometimes say the right things when you need it.
—Melissa, white woman of high SES

Infertility is not solely a medical condition that takes place in the confines of doctors' offices, as past literature and stereotypes have implied. It occurs within the context of women's everyday lives. Indeed, infertility "is not something in which there are 'social factors'; it is itself a profoundly social phenomenon" (Schneider and Conrad 1983, 227). It is therefore important to investigate how and why social and cultural factors shape the infertility experience. *Social* context in particular is especially influential in shaping an individual's understanding of and reaction to childbearing difficulties (Miall 1986).

Most infertility research does not study the social basis of infertility; it objectifies it as a medical issue (Greil, Slauson-Blevins, and McQuillan 2010). As infertility becomes medicalized, medical institutions inform the context in which it is experienced. In turn, the sufferers of infertility are transformed into "patients" (Greil 1991). This is especially true for infertility research, wherein the majority of studies recruit participants from medical clinics, resulting in samples composed entirely of patients. Recruiting participants in such a manner, while convenient, results in homogenous samples of white, affluent women. Doing so leads to facile generalizations of infertility experiences, generalizations that diminish the importance of context by treating the infertility experience as invariant or taking the dominant group's infertility experiences as a proxy for the experiences of all women (Kirkman and Rosenthal 1999). But experiences of infertility do vary; there are many "infertilities" (Sandelowski 1993). Infertility does not discriminate along race or class lines, yet the context in which it is lived depends upon such factors, and thus the experience of infertility varies accordingly.

To understand how social class shapes the experience of infertility, researchers must follow two recommendations. First, as sociologist Patricia Hill Collins (1994, 5) suggests, emphasizing the "social base" of phenomena, such as infertility and reproduction, requires a focus on *variation* rather than on universal. Following Collins's recommendation, I show how experiences vary among women of different social classes and reveal infertility as a unique process that cannot and should not be generalized among all women. Second, as women researchers of color have noted, it is necessary to place marginalized women's experiences at the center of analysis in order to "recontextualize," or discover different contexts for, infertility; when white, higher-class women's experiences remain prominent, race and class become invisible. Comparing women of high and low SES allows several dimensions of context to "stand out in stark relief" (Collins 1994, 61): differences in peer context, marital norms, social support, and disclosure practices expose the social basis of infertility and how it is constructed according to dominant notions of race, class, and gender.

Stereotypes of Infertility

Despite sharing an equally high prevalence of infertility, poor women and women of color are constructed as hyperfertile, while infertility is stereotyped as primarily affecting white, middle- and upper-class women (Chandra, Copen, and Stephen 2013; Kelly 2010; Marsh and Ronner 1996). In this study women of both high and low SES internalize those inaccurate stereotypes that shape their experiences of infertility. Rachelle, a black woman of low SES in her late twenties, describes her experience:

> RACHELLE: Mm (pauses), 'cuz like pretty much brought up when I ever heard about someone not being able to have a child, they would always been white. I had never personally met or interacted with an African American woman that couldn't.... I said, "Why did I have that image in my head?"
> ANN: Right.
> RACHELLE: I don't know. I really—I think just because as far as like TV or books or magazines, every time there was an issue, I always would see a white woman.
> ANN: Mm-hm. Yeah. And do you know of any black women who are having issues?
> RACHELLE: Personally, I don't . . . Mm-mm, I don't know of any personally.

The image of infertility as a white woman's issue was normalized for Rachelle, in the sense that she "does not know" why she conjures up such a picture when thinking about infertility. Moreover, the media perpetuates the stereotype and infertility's (seeming) absence from Rachelle's own context. In my interviews with women of low SES, references to media were commonplace. The participants frequently mentioned shows such as *Jon and Kate Plus 8, Oprah, The Baby Story,* and the Lifetime Channel when discussing infertility. Bonnie, a black woman of low SES working as a lab assistant, gives one such example:

ANN: Do you know anybody who's had difficulty?

BONNIE: No. Only what I've seen on television.... You know, when I do think about it, I do, yeah, about Oprah she did. But that's on fertilities and then trying to get pregnant but as far as like, you know, like a show actually why or information out—I mean it may be out there. I don't think it's easily accessible—you know, to find out, "Okay, what is it that women at these certain age, demographics or whatever can't have kids?"

Bonnie actively seeks out information about infertility from shows such as *Oprah*. Her only referent for what the "infertile person" looks like is through the media, which typically reifies it as occurring among the dominant group: white women of high SES. Like Rachelle, Bonnie does not personally know anyone who has had childbearing difficulty, which compounds her notion of infertility as occurring among women of other demographics.

Similarly, Nadia, a white woman of high SES, internalizes the norm of infertility as a white, wealthy woman's issue:

I think that a lot of the minority classes have less problems with infertility and it's bad enough when you're going through it as Indian or white but what about when you're in a race where nobody has that problem?... Now whether that doesn't necessarily translate to fertility problems. And same with white women I think have a higher percentage of problems than Hispanic or white—or—or black or Asian. I think it would be worse in the other cultures. In fact, my friend without the fallopian tubes is black and she doesn't know anybody that is going through what she does. I have a friend who is Chinese. It's among the lowest infertility rates and she doesn't know anybody who is going through what she is, who is—who is Chinese. I think then socioeconomically also it would be much more difficult.... I'm like, "Wow, we're lucky because at least even though my insurance only covers fifty, at least that's part of it and at least I have a job."... You know. You know, at least I am in a job where I can go in to work a little late because I had to go in to my fertility clinic.... I think it would be a lot more difficult depending on—because there is nothing. Like if I didn't have the funds to do this myself, I'd be—I'd—I'd be out of luck.

Nadia believes that the experience of infertility would be different for women of different races and economic circumstances. She has internalized the stereotype of infertility as an issue among women of her demographic group: white and high-income women. Additionally, that stereotype is perpetuated by her friends who belong to marginalized racial groups and who also believe that infertility is a white woman's issue because they do not know of anyone of their race who is infertile. Perhaps most important, Nadia highlights how an individual's social location and the stereotypes and ideologies surrounding that location shape her experiences of infertility.

In addition to internalizing the stereotype as to who is infertile, the participants internalized the gendered idea that all women mother, as explored in chapter 1. The women believed their desire to mother was innate and a normal part of womanhood. As a result, all the women in the study felt alone and marginalized. For women of low SES, however, the belief that infertility only occurs among white women of higher classes compounded these feelings. In other words, women of high SES are marginalized within motherhood and thus womanhood, whereas women of low SES are marginalized within both motherhood *and* infertility itself. Women of low SES must challenge two dominant stereotypes: all women are mothers, and all infertile women are higher class.

"I Was Different": The Peer Context of Infertility

In exploring the participants' social surroundings, I examine how such stereotypes play out and are influenced by the circumstances of women's lives. Other research has studied such effects. In a study of teenage pregnancy, researchers found that the teenagers' interactions with others were shaped by stereotypes of teen pregnancy that portray it as a negative life experience and identity (Brubaker and Wright 2006). Infertility is also intimately connected with social functioning and relationships. Indeed, one study found that infertile women struggle with socializing in a pronatalist culture. The women are confronted with "coercive social exchanges" in which they are constantly questioned about their childlessness (Sandelowski and Jones 1986, 174). But as I demonstrate with the following findings, such effects vary depending upon one's social location. Earlier childbearing, higher frequency of children, and less ability to map out their life goals uniquely shape the low SES women's responses to infertility.

Reflective of the internalization of the stereotype of infertility as a white, wealthy woman's issue, the women of low SES do not know many others with infertility. When asked if she knew of anyone who was infertile, Tiffany, a black woman of low SES working part-time at McDonald's, answers: "Mm-mm . . . Nope. I sure do not. No. Like everybody in my family has at least one. Everybody." For the few women of low SES who do know someone with childbearing difficulties, the person is typically someone at a distance with whom they cannot relate. Judy, a white woman of low SES in her late thirties, describes her "distant cousin" who experienced infertility: "I have—I have a distant cousin and she had fertility issues but she's like really her and her husband are really overweight like they weigh like 500. She weighs like 5—4 or 500 pounds and she's allowed to have gastric bypass. [The doctors] just approved her but they like spent every last dime they had for in vitro because they kept trying and trying and I don't know if it had to do with her weight." Judy only knows of this one "distant" relative who has had childbearing difficulties. She is unable to relate to her cousin's experience; Judy cannot afford IVF, and she does not consider herself to have the same weight problems. Instead, Judy distances herself from her cousin's fertility troubles by focusing on those differences.

In addition to not knowing anyone well who has experienced infertility or childbearing problems, the women of low SES live in a context in which most of their peers have children, which furthers their feelings of marginalization. For instance, Donna, a black woman of low SES, wanted to "get on the bandwagon" because "everybody was having 'em and everybody was getting together, you know, having kid parties and stuff so it kind of made them—me feel a little left out." Candace, a black woman of low SES, echoes Donna's feelings: "I just always thought something was wrong, I was different. I knew I was different because all of my friends had babies. And you'd see 'em in the grocery store with their children and different things. So I knew something was different (laughs)."

These feelings of "difference" may stem from the strong focus on motherhood in poor communities. As Ebony, a black woman of low SES, explains to me at a community center, motherhood is the primary identity, role, and action for women in her demographic group: "But then it's more like my friends and their—them having a lot of kids, it's like, 'Okay, we have kids. That's what we do.' Like, you know . . . to have kids was just the norm. That's the norm like, you know, you might have a kid by this guy, this guy, which is—that's not classy or that's very nasty, they call it or people say it. But some people do it to start a family or do whatever they—whatever plan they have is why they do it. You know." Having children is what women in Ebony's community "do"; having children is the "norm" and thus the focus of their life goals because other rewarding activities, such as occupations or hobbies, are less attainable.

Without a variety of life events and occurrences to discuss, women of low SES have difficulty identifying with or interacting with their peers. Jocelyn, a black woman of low SES, explains that she does not "have [anything] in common with [her friends] anymore." Ruby, a white woman of low SES, further elaborates on the issue:

> It's—I don't feel socially accepted sometimes because all my friends now have children or are settling down and have children. None of them have problems I guess. And I have quite a few friends. . . . But I don't feel socially accepted in any way. . . . I can't bond with the adults [at work] because I just can't. I have— and I ha—what (crying)—what interests do I really have to them if they're— have families? I have—me and my husband have barely any (pauses) friends work- work-related and I—other than high school friends that I have, we don't have any friends that we can go out and go, "Let's go have a drink because we have interests. You know, because we have families. We—we can't do that." We tried joining a bowling league right here and trying that and that fizzled out. You know. We either are too young for the people or we don't have kids and we're not family. We're oddball. It just—I just—I just—a horrible thing.

Ruby feels that she and her husband are "oddballs" because they cannot fit in socially. People their age all have children and those without children tend to be too old to share similar interests. Earlier childbearing norms in which women of low SES have children at younger ages leave fewer childless couples in middle age (Martinez, Daniels, and Chandra 2012).

The earlier childbearing norms among those of economically disadvantaged settings cause even the participants who were eventually able to have children to feel abnormal. Their fertility difficulties delayed their childbearing, leaving them older at first birth than their peers. Barbara, a forty-four-year-old black woman of low SES, reflects:

> Sometimes you feel I guess it would be just left out. You know, when all of your other friends because my—my peers, my friends, my college friends and everything, their kids are now, you know, at least—at the—at the very least,

in their tee—in their teens. But, you know, most of them have children who are adults. You know, when I say adults I mean eighteen plus years old. So and here I am with a two-year-old. You know, so, you know, it—it's a—it's a lonely place to be because again, you don't have a lot of parents but not a lot of parents around you who are in the same place. . . . I don't have a lot of friends who have young children.

Barbara is "lonely" because most of her friends have older children while she is the mother of a two-year-old. Laura, a forty-year-old white woman of low SES, reiterates Barbara's concerns: "So that hurt seeing the family, you know, my nieces having kids when I should have been having 'em. Like now my sister, she's raising her grandson and he's two years older than Molly, you know, so she's raising her grandchild and I'm raising my daughter." Laura "should have been having" children earlier according to the norms of those around her, but her infertility made it impossible to do so. As a result, she has difficulty relating to family members who are at different life stages.

In addition to early childbearing norms and fewer attainable and identifiable goals, the low-income women's norm of "redemptive mothering"—the belief that motherhood will cause them to mature—shapes their infertility experience (McMahon 1995). Tanya, a white woman of low SES, says: "My friends growing—growing up and doing the same—not the same thing but—but finally had a—a way to go, you know, in life instead of just partying or shopping or hanging out or whatever." Tanya was jealous of her friends' ability to "grow up" after having children. She felt that her childlessness prevented her from achieving full adulthood.

Candace, a black woman of low SES, expresses the same concerns: "All of my friends growing up were having babies and I mean that could have been good for me but I didn't think that at the time. They was having babies, moving out of their moms' houses, getting apartments. So I moved down out of my mom's house and got with my boyfriend. But I always still wanted a baby. And I think it affected me in some ways in my life. I'm still a big kid. I look younger for my age and I act younger." To Candace, her friends were able to grow up as a result of having children. She seems to yearn for their more "adult" lifestyle and believes that her childlessness causes her to remain a "big kid." Her statement also reflects other social norms in disadvantaged communities: "all" of her friends have children, and they had them at younger ages when they were still living with their mothers.

Given differing norms in their communities, such as the norm of delaying childbearing, the infertility experiences of women of high SES diverge from those discussed among women of low SES. Like their poorer counterparts, women of high SES do not know of many others with infertility, which attests to the silence and invisibility of infertility as a social problem. Unlike women of low SES, however, women of high SES are able to relate to those that they do know or the images they see because the stereotype of infertility matches their demographic characteristics. Sarah explains this connection:

> I mean I heard of people that I kind of knew growing up and my mother would say, you know, "So-and-So had to go to wherever and have *in vitro*." And I was like, "Oh, wow." You know, but there was no—no, I didn't know anybody. Nobody close. And now there's only—it's only two really. The one I work with and the one I used to work with who I don't really talk to but she and I had one conversation about it recently. Because another friend who I do stay in touch with had said, "You and Jen should talk" so we just got on the phone one night and talked for an hour and she actually had gone to the exact same doctor that I am seeing now so we had very similar—but no, I didn't know anybody. This was like really foreign because I really didn't think that it would ever happen to me.

Even though Sarah did not know anyone "close" to her who struggled with infertility, she was aware of women in similar circumstances who experienced difficulties in childbearing. Acquaintances of Sarah's mother and friends provided Sarah with an image of the characteristics of women who experience infertility although she did not know these women well. Indeed, she had "very similar" experiences to a friend of a friend so could relate well enough to her to "talk for an hour." This contrasts with Judy's experience of distancing herself from her obese cousin.

While the women of low SES felt like they did not fit in with their peers due to early childbearing norms and restricted life goals, women of high SES felt marginalized because they failed to conform to the dominant norm of pronatalism. Nadia, a program manager, reflects on this marginalization:

> I, you know, I have never had mine . . . and it's really hard because it's always around you. You know, it's like it's not like you can avoid it. You know? It's

not like you can shield yourself from it. You go to work and people are talking about kids and you turn on the TV. People, you know, there's kids' commercials, you know, you drive down the freeway and there is—I just today saw, you know, about this hospital being great for, you know, delivering babies and I mean it's all—everywhere and especially in the last few years it's fashionable to have kids. Now it's the thing. I mean ten to fifteen years ago you didn't see it, you know, on *People* magazine. Now it's the thing to do.

Pronatalism is embedded in Nadia's surroundings. Billboards, television, and magazines all display children, families, and mothers to the point where Nadia cannot "avoid it." Nadia's race and socioeconomic status define her as part of the dominant group that is typically reflected in the media. Unlike women of low SES on the margins of motherhood, who refer to not fitting in with their peers, Nadia expresses the sense of not fitting in with society at large.

Additionally, the norms present in higher-class contexts allow the women of high SES the ability to still relate to and fit in with their peers. For instance, rather than having children at younger ages, women of high SES live in an environment in which delayed childbearing is normal. This allows many of the high-income participants, unlike the poor and working-class participants who found themselves isolated, to continue to have many childless friends. As Sarah, a white woman of high SES, states: "I still have quite a few [friends] that don't [have children]. People that just haven't worked it into their schedule to start trying or they're a little younger or I have—we hang out with quite a few people who are much older, some not married and some that were never able to have kids for other reasons. So yeah, there are lots of people that we hang out with that don't have kids, too. So yeah, I don't get that so much 'cuz they're not constantly in my face. Yeah, so I guess that's good." Sarah, unlike Ruby, does not feel like an "oddball" because she has friends who do not have children. This is due to different life-course trajectories and "schedules" in which examples of delayed childbearing, delayed marriage, and perhaps more voluntary childlessness are present in Sarah's high SES environment. Life goals beyond having children, coupled with the ability to control and choose one's actions, such as reproduction, are present in economically advantaged contexts and thus differentially shape their experiences of infertility.

"The Only Type of Relationship I Need": The Marital Context of Infertility

Not only do women of low and high SES have different peer norms, but they also have different marital and partnering norms as well, which ultimately shape their infertility experiences. Past research (for example, Greil, Leitko, and Porter 1988) has shown the significant impact of infertility on relationships, either making couples stronger or tearing them apart; but the effects are reciprocal: the relationship itself affects the infertility experience. The interviews reveal that women in committed partnerships are better able to cope with infertility through the support they receive from their partners. Because most women of low SES, particularly black women, are not in a relationship or are in fluctuating relationships in which monogamy and long-term commitment are typically absent, they lack the social support that could help mitigate some of infertility's negative effects (Hill 2004; Lundquist, Budig, and Curtis 2009).

Poor women and women of color marry less frequently than their white, higher-class counterparts (Hill 2004). This trend is reflected in the study sample: all white women of high SES were married compared to only 19 percent of black women of low SES and 60 percent of white women of low SES. For black women and women of low SES, marriage is not an important prerequisite to having children (Blum and Deussen 1996; Edin and Kefalas 2005). Indeed, more black women have children when they are not married. One reason for this is that children take precedence over marriage in the black (poor) context by providing more stable and permanent relationships than marriage. Sociologist Jennifer Lundquist and colleagues (2009) found that childlessness is actually associated with marriage among blacks. Mikela, a black woman of low SES, demonstrates such thinking when I asked her why she did not believe marriage was important:

> Because marriage don't work out. . . . The only thing that's stable is their kid that's going to be there for real is their kid. If you guys have a kid, that's it. That's what ya'll work through. If ya'll can love that kid and love each other, then that's fine. But you don't have to be married. I don't believe that . . . I don't believe you have to have to be married to have kids because marriage don't work. . . . Marriage don't last. But that baby there . . . that's last—that's important. You've got to build that. That's the only type of relationship I need

and if you can't give me that respectful type of relationship with my kids, then just don't come around.

Many women of low SES echoed and extended Mikela's claim that babies were important to gain stability in life because marriages "don't last."

Fear of infidelity was the crux of marital instability in the black women's accounts. Tiffany, a black woman of low SES, explains:

ANN: Is marriage important, do you think?

TIFFANY: Mm-mm. I'm not getting married.

ANN: Why not?

TIFFANY: Mm-mm. I don't like that. 'Cuz marriage is supposed to be a bond between two people and not two people and like some outside people. Mm-mm . . . I would rather just say you're boyfriend/girlfriend, whatever and just keep it like that. We can have a common law marriage but we ain't got to be married like that. I—I'm not into the marriage thing. . . . And then I look at a lot of marriages now and like how the women feel when their husband is off and doing their own thing and stuff like that. That's why I'd rather just stay your girlfriend and we can keep it like that. At least I know with being your girlfriend, I already know you're going to step up. When I'm your wife, that's something you shouldn't do.

For women of low SES like Tiffany, infidelity is frequently not looked down upon in nonmarital relationships, such as boyfriend/girlfriend partnerships, but in marriage it is "something you shouldn't do." Therefore, many women, fearing that infidelity will continue, oppose marriage.

A few of the black participants were married, going against the cultural norms. This typically occurred among more religious women, such as Josie, a hospital worker. She states:

I wanted to be definitely married first. That's—my family, like I said, they're very religious but I didn't see myself getting married at twenty-two but it happened and it was a good thing. I have always wanted to be married, to have a family of my own that I kind of like took care of, you know, me and my husband or whatever. And I definitely wanted to be married before I had kids. Growing up in high school you would see girls pregnant and not that it was like a shame but I just didn't want that for myself. I just wanted to be married and, you know, make it through high school without having any kids, you know. So that was like my biggest thing.

Josie was surrounded by young women having children out of wedlock; however, true to her religious beliefs and upbringing, she did not want that for herself and considered it an accomplishment that she "made it through high school without having any kids."

Although more white women of low SES were married than black women in the study, 40 percent of white women of low SES remained unmarried. A convergence of marginalized and dominant norms in low-income communities may contribute to the diversity in marriage rates among white women of low SES (Harding 2007). Jodi, a white woman of low SES, describes the various kinds of partnerships that take place among the economically disadvantaged:

ANN: How about—how about for most of your friends? Are most of them in like stable relationships when they have kids or no?

JODI: Mm, yes and no. Like Miranda—Miranda, you know, Miranda has— Johnny ... but [they are] no longer [together]. Let's see. Deanna, yes, she is. She's married. All of her babies have the same father. (Pauses) I mean there's just so many I can't even count—that have either different baby daddies or not—or with other people or—or are just single.

White participants of low SES are surrounded by women who are in committed relationships, casual relationships, and no relationships at all. Such heterogeneity of norms results in more diverse attitudes about marriage among white women of low SES.

For some low-income white women, understandings of marriage mirrored those of black women of low SES. Jackie, a socially anxious, white woman of low SES, describes how nonmarital childbearing is the norm in her context: "Everybody (pauses)—everybody I know got—had—got their baby before they were married, you know, or got pregnant before they were married. Well, you know, most people." Similarly, Judy, an unemployed white woman of low SES, describes how she does not want to marry for fear of infidelity: "But as for a lifetime relationship, I'm not—I don't know. Do you know what I mean? I don't even know—I don't think I want that with really anybody. . . . I just don't trust men and—not at all . . . because I've been cheated on before. So."

While Jackie and Judy convey their reasons for not getting married, several white women of low SES in the study were married. For the majority of the married participants of low SES, however, it was not that *they* believed marriage was important for having children, but rather that others held such a belief. This may indicate shifting familial norms among low-income white individuals: the women's parents believed marriage was necessary for parenting, yet the women themselves did not share such a belief. Nicole, a white woman of low SES, reflects on this phenomenon:

> I—I didn't want to disappoint my parents, you know, having a child and not married. That would have devastated them, you know, so I was always looking for boyfriends that would marry me, you know, just so that I could have a kid. You know, then I got married and then he doesn't (laughing) want to have them. So yeah, I kind of screwed up on that one (both laughing). Yeah. But, you know, 'cuz that would have just absolutely broken their hearts. So, you know, I always tried to—that's why I stayed on the birth control so that I wouldn't, you know, upset them and stuff, so.

Nicole did not believe marriage was necessary for having children, but she chose to marry so as not to "disappoint" her parents. She is now in a very unhappy "open" marriage and lives with her boyfriend on the weekends.

Juxtaposed against these diverse views of marriage and childbearing among low-income white women were the highly consistent views of marital norms among white women of high SES. All the high-income participants were married, and all believed marriage was a prerequisite to having children. As Linda, a plainspoken white woman of high SES, elaborates: "I'm not extremely like it wasn't about religion or anything like that. I always wanted to be married. I didn't think about it like I say in great de—great detail. I just sort of, you know, planned it out that way like get married and then have kids, you know, don't get pregnant or you know what I mean." Linda "didn't think" about being married before having kids because such a norm was unquestioned in her community. As the privileged environment allows, Linda planned her life-course to adhere to the typical trajectory.

The importance of following the proper sequence of life stages is further demonstrated by Iris, a white woman of high SES: "Yeah, well, we—I didn't want us to start trying until after we got married because I wanted to—because we got married fifteen days after I graduated from graduate school and so I didn't want to be pregnant during graduate school and I didn't want to be pregnant and during the wedding. So we didn't really start before that. So as soon as we got married, we started and we knew that that was how it was going to be." Dominant norms define a (good) family as a (heterosexual) married couple with child(ren). This constructed ideal is so taken-for-granted in the typical life plans of women of high SES that they cannot articulate why it is necessary to be married before having children; rather, they simply "knew that that was how it was going to be."

Adhering to the normative order of life stages was the reason some participants of high SES were struggling with their fertility. Waiting for marriage before childbearing caused some of the women to experience age-related infertility. Colleen, a white woman of high SES, is one such participant:

> I didn't like it. Well, it's not that I didn't like being single. I enjoyed my single years. I had a fantastic job, I traveled, I, you know, I had great friends, I took trips. But I really wanted to be married and have a family. So that was—that was very, very hard for me and I knew I wanted kids and so, you know, the older I got, it got harder and harder and, you know, I tried not to be bitter. But it was tough because all of my friends were doing, you know, doing my thing on my timeline. You know, they had all gotten married, you know, I was the maid of honor in like five different weddings. And, you know, then I was godmother to how many different kids and throwing all of these baby showers and I mean that was even before I knew I was going to have trouble.

Despite wanting to be married, Colleen did not find the right partner until later in life and was thus not able to adhere to the typical high SES "time line." The precedence of marriage before children led to delayed childbearing and ensuing infertility.

The differences in marital norms between the socioeconomic groups led to differences in the women's infertility experiences. Given their lower rates of marriage, women of low SES, particularly black women, did not receive spousal support for their childbearing difficulties. Moreover, because of the more on again/off again relationships in low-income communities, the women of low SES who were in relationships feared that their boyfriends would leave them if they found out about their fertility problems. Angie, a black woman of low SES, explains:

> ANN: Why do you think that your current boyfriend might not stay with you if you tell him that you can't have children?
>
> ANGIE: Because it's like—because it's part of like—I don't know—well, like to me, it's part of growing [a family]. If—if you can't, you know, like grow with me and us have a wonderful life, what are you here for? . . . We can be together until we're old but I mean I know—I know he wants to have kids. I want to have kids. But me telling him that I can't have kids, I just feel he'll leave. . . . Because a guy always want to, you know, plant their seed and, you know, they always want to have a kid.

Angie, like many women of low SES, had not told her boyfriend about her childbearing difficulties. Because she was not married, her boyfriend could easily leave her to "plant his seed" elsewhere. Such fears are class- and race-based, but they also represent gendered understandings that the ultimate "purpose" of women is to reproduce—"what else are you here for?"

Evidence of the additional support marriage provides to infertile women is apparent among women of low SES who were married. Josie, a black woman of low SES, reflects on such support: "[My husband] is like the best. He's—he's totally like, 'Okay. It's okay. If we can't have our own kids, we'll adopt kids. It's not a big deal.' You know, he's just like—one day I thought that I kind of was pregnant and I thought I was having symptoms and I am just completely in tears and I didn't tell him what was wrong with me and he's like—when I finally did tell him, he was like, 'I figured that was what was wrong with you.' And he kind of stayed home with me from work. He's like totally supportive. Just 100 percent." Roberta, a white woman of low SES, describes similar experiences with her husband: "You know, honestly [my husband] was so supportive and even since then when I get down about it or whatever and I talk to him about it, he just, you know, 'Honey, it's all right. It wasn't meant to be. It's not that, you know, it's not a problem.'" Roberta's husband serves as a source of social support with whom she can talk about her struggles. He also provides her with words of advice and reassurance.

One of the most consistent comments of women of high SES concerned the significant support they received from their husbands. Only one of the seventeen higher-class women's relationships was disrupted to the point of separation because of infertility, and even they reconciled and are now a "success." Stephanie, a white woman of high SES, demonstrates this high level of support:

> Yeah, I don't—[my husband] never was negative about it. He was very positive, which I'm sure played a huge role in me feeling that way. . . . I think if it had been any other way, he would have, you know, I would have felt worse. Even after the fact that we knew that it probably had nothing to do with his body and it had something to do with mine, he still was very supportive. We joked about it, you know, in fun but we could because it was just the two of us. It wasn't anyone else joking about it. But then it stayed there tabled and it—and we just moved forward. And so he was a positive influence.

Stephanie's husband's optimism "played a huge role" in her coping with infertility. In fact, his "positive influence" allowed them to "move forward" in their childbearing journey. Becca's husband was a similar positive influence on her infertility experience. She reflects on his support when she states, "And I sometimes accuse him of having a little playbook on the other side of the bed that he looks up the answers to because they're all so perfect."

Rather than tear relationships apart, as Angie feared, infertility often brought couples of high SES closer together. Nan, a highly educated, white woman of high SES, demonstrates this point:

> In truth [infertility] has drawn us closer. Much closer. Just we've had to really kind of cling to each other and, you know, pouring out our sorrows to each other or mostly me but him, too. Just it drew us much closer going through—going through something like this together. . . . It just, you know, like I mentioned before, it always felt like it was just something that we were experiencing together and it wasn't—it wasn't like a me against him kind of thing. So it was just something that we went through together and we weathered the ups and downs of it together and it drew us closer. You know, I had to learn to communicate with each other on a deeper level and how to comfort each other and be patient with each other.

Although it is not the case for many infertile couples, in this study the childbearing struggles experienced by the women of high SES seemed to benefit relationships rather than hurt them. Not knowing many others who have gone through infertility, couples relied on each other to cope with their difficulties. When that support is neither present nor permanent, as is the case for many women of low SES, particularly black women, the infertility experience is a lonelier journey.

"I Don't Have Much Support": Social Support Beyond Marriage

Beyond spousal and partner support, other forms of support shape infertility experiences. The participants' socioeconomic status shapes the presence and prevalence of various types of support. Many women of low SES do not have the resources or access to certain types of support, such as therapy. By contrast, women of high SES have not only the economic means to pay for such support but also the knowledge of how to find it.

When discussing their support systems, women of low SES never mentioned friends or peers. The absence of such support may result from the feeling among women of low SES that they could no longer relate to or fit in with their peers due to earlier childbearing norms and less accessible alternative life goals in their communities. In addition to losing the support of friends, women of low SES in the study discussed a lack of support from family. As Ruby, a white woman of low SES, explains:

> So and everybody just—I know that's the reason they cater to [my sister] because she has children. They—and she throws and she gets her way and I'm just like, "That is so unfair." And everybody will deny it. But it is—my husband sees it so. And outsiders see it. It's just my family's in denial. Oh, it just—it pisses me off sometimes . . . so. And no one—no one thinks to call me first about something. They call my sister . . . so. It's—that's—that's probably like the worst of it all is no one will remember you because you didn't have a family socialness going on. So yeah, that's probably the worst.

Without children, Ruby does not have "family socialness" so she is "forgotten" by her family. She believes that her sister receives more attention and money from her parents because she has children. Ruby's childlessness marginalizes her socially as well as economically and personally with her family.

Although participants of low SES infrequently mentioned social support, some cited religion as helping them get through their difficulties. Angie, a black woman of low SES, states: "My pastor [provides the most emotional support]. . . . Yeah, we prayed about it. He told me, you know, 'When it's time, it's time (laughing).' Okay, it's God's work. . . . He's really I mean giving me good support. But I haven't actually gotten down in detail of, you know, me not having or being able to have kids. But he knows something is wrong and he's just not saying anything." Angie's pastor provides her with more support than any other person, yet it is indirect support because she has not told him about her struggles with childbearing. Moreover, black women typically do not disclose their infertility to others. In the absence of alternatives, the mere presence of someone who knows that "something is wrong" provides Angie with some peace of mind.

A few of the women of low SES turned to the Internet for support. As Tamara, a black woman of low SES in her mid-twenties, explains: "So I'd rather blog about it . . . then speak about it and maybe someone else besides myself who had—who's experiencing the same thing I am going through and you've got to lift yourself up no matter what family or friends they say to you, you can always do it, you know." Blogging allows Tamara to relate to other women like her who are experiencing childbearing difficulties. For women of low SES who do not receive much support from friends or family and know of few other infertile women, the Internet provides a way to "lift yourself up" in spite of such conditions.

The women of low SES offer several explanations for their lack of support for their fertility troubles. Donna, a black woman of low SES, explains that it is due to her reluctance to disclose her infertility: "No, [I don't have much support] because like I said (laughs), don't nobody know. So. And then they think I like not having kids. So no, it's kind of like that. I have to like run in the corner a little bit and cry it without and then everybody do but. It don't affect me that much like it had been maybe within the last year or so. But yeah, so it hadn't been that—that much of a problem. But no, socially, no, I'm a loner (laughs) a little bit." As mentioned previously, the majority of the participants of low SES do not tell many people of their childbearing difficulties. Donna is a "loner" perhaps as a result of her childlessness, but from her story it is clear that she is struggling emotionally with infertility. Rather than recognizing Donna's childbearing troubles, people "think [she] likes not having kids." Her statement suggests that she has

internalized both the stereotype of infertility as exclusively a white, affluent woman's problem and the motherhood mandate that treats having children as normal and childlessness as abnormal.

Women of low SES also attribute their lack of support to their socioeconomic status. Mikela, a thirty-year-old black woman of low SES,
believes that "somebody that's either getting help or wealthy enough or—
economically speaking . . . —like have a good support system that helps
you that way. You know? That it matters." According to Mikela, money
"matters" because having a "good support system" depends on economics.

Rachelle, a black woman of low SES, concurs: "Maybe like financial
options 'cuz like I know a lot of those fertility clinics and things like that
cost a lot of money, you know, and—I don't know—maybe—I think people probably do have more support than I did. I don't know. At least somebody you could talk to or something." Rachelle did not have anyone to talk
to about her childbearing difficulties. She could not even talk with a physician because she lacked access to health care, which she attributes to her
limited economic circumstances.

In addition to monetary restrictions, low SES women's lack of knowledge about available resources and support places them at a disadvantage.
Formal support groups for infertility abound, but, because of their market-
ing strategies, location, and focus on medical treatment, they are predomi-
nately composed of white, higher-class women. Angie, a black woman of
low SES, describes her lack of knowledge about such groups: "To not have
no support is how this is crazy. I haven't ever even heard of any groups out
there, you know, for people like me. And because there will probably—I
don't know—I never even thought anything like this before but my friend
has and it was crazy. But kidnapping—it would probably cut down a lot
of kidnappings and, you know, people trying to take, you know, people's
kids." Angie has not "ever even heard of any groups out there." Angie wants
more support but does not know where to find it.

Women of high SES, in contrast, not only know about support resources
available, but they utilize them to their full advantage. Colleen, a white
woman of high SES, describes attending RESOLVE, the largest national
support organization for infertility:

> And we were going to RESOLVE meetings. . . . They were great meetings
> for us. It was good to have other people to talk to who got it. Who got how
> it controlled your life. Who got how you could never make plans and how

tiring it was to go to—for appointments, you know, driving to the university and parking in that Godawful structure to go in for a blood draw. You know, I mean they got it. And it was good for resources to talk about doctors and to talk about pharmacies. "What's the best pharmacy to get your drugs?" Because, you know, certainly a rural pharmacy's not going to have a full, you know, selection of Gonal-F and all of these other things you have to take. And so it was great from that standpoint and it was great to hear what other people went through because it really gave us things to talk about. . . . But so from that standpoint, you know, those meetings were great for us. And we, you know, I wouldn't say we became friends with those people. We—it was very nice to be there and we would always go out afterward, you know, for whatever.

Attending RESOLVE provided support to Colleen on many levels. It provided her with access to other women in her situation who could "relate" to her experiences, and they socialized together. It also gave her resources, such as access to medical knowledge. Women of low SES already have limited access to such resources. Not knowing about or participating in groups such as RESOLVE further exacerbates their lack of resources, and thus the class divide persists.

Women of high SES also receive professional support such as psychotherapy that is economically not an option for women of low SES. Iris, a white woman of high SES, explains her experience: "Yeah, yeah, did I have support. I think I had a lot of support when I was going through it and when I made the choice to—to do [IVF] and we were like on board and doing the drugs, there was definitely a lot of support then. . . . But also my therapist—a couples therapist we had at the time was—also happened to be a therapist for the clinic, the IVF clinic. So she was very aware of the emotions that I might be going through . . . so she was really helpful." Iris was the one participant of high SES whose relationship suffered because of fertility problems; however, her ability to access therapy allowed the couple to reconcile, and they are currently thriving. This same therapist was able to provide Iris with emotional support for her childbearing difficulties.

Because they often knew other women without children, and because they shared common interests outside of mothering with women who had children, women of high SES maintained more friendships than did the women of low SES I have described. Thus, peers were a strong support system for high SES women in this study. Stephanie, a white substitute teacher of high SES, elaborates on the support she received from her friends: "I do [think I had support]. I do. Because, interesting enough, like when some-one would be pregnant, the closest of close friends would know—they would say, 'Are you okay?' Just checking in. Not to dwell on it, not to make it more than what it was but just making sure." Stephanie's friends were able to prevent her from slipping into despair by consistently "checking in" when necessary. They knew what triggered her emotions around childbear-ing issues and "made sure" that she was "okay" in their presence.

Similarly, Melissa, a white librarian of high SES, describes her support: "So I think we've got a lot of support, which is nice. . . . You know, people that we can rely on not to judge and just be supportive and sometimes say the right things when you need it. So and then I also have friends that are absolutely against having children themselves and they're like, 'If you want to, that's fine but I don't really—it doesn't even appeal to me' (laughs). Okay. So it's kind of—for me, I've got a lot of people that have different opinions and so it's kind of nice." Melissa's statement reiterates the diver-sity of high SES women's friendships. In contrast to "all" of the low SES women's friends having children, the delayed childbearing, voluntary childlessness, and accessibility to more diverse life goals of women of high SES allows them to be able to relate to others. Moreover, for the women of high SES those friendships provide a support network that is missing from the experiences of economically disadvantaged women. Like some of the women of low SES, however, a few of the women of high SES turned to religion for support. Nan, a white woman of high SES, "had two priests that [she] would talk to frequently who were friends and [she] could talk to them in kind of spiritual counseling."

Despite the numerous resources and individuals available to support women of high SES with their fertility struggles, some of the participants believe this support is insufficient. Nadia, a white woman of high SES, explains:

> We don't really—there's really no formal support for women going through this. It's, you know, if you were going through a divorce, your friends rally around you. If you're going through a death, there's a funeral and there's clo-sure and you move on. With infertility, it's like month after month you're almost— . . . It's like you're mourning a loss every month that doesn't happen. It's almost like the loss of a child that never was. It's almost like mourning a death and one thing I did read is that they say that going through infertility is like more traumatic than, you know, is as traumatic or more than any other

thing they have measured on a trauma scale in life. But yet, what do they have out there? RESOLVE.

Given the "traumatic" and ever-present experience of infertility, Nadia yearns for more support than she receives. The lack of a concrete event, like divorce, or a definitive ending, like death, makes infertility unique, and thus it requires more and different support than is currently available. Medicalizing infertility objectifies the experience, and its emotional, personal, and social repercussions go unnoticed, leaving the women who experience it with limited options, regardless of their social location.

Talking About Childbearing Difficulties

Infertility is a "hidden" problem, in that it must be verbalized for others to know it exists. Whether the participants revealed their infertility to others depended on their social location. Rates of disclosure differed by race and class because cultural practices influenced the likelihood that participants' would discuss their childbearing difficulties. These differences, in turn, further increased variation in experiences of infertility.

Women of low SES, particularly black women, do not tell many people, if any, about their childbearing difficulties. Not talking about their experiences furthers the stereotype that infertility is a white, wealthy woman's issue and maintains the feelings of isolation and loneliness that a marginalized group experiences. For black women, however, not discussing personal issues is a cultural practice. This silencing may stem from the "strength mandate" imposed on black women, which implies that they are "less than a woman" if they show signs of weakness. Sociologist Shirley Hill (2009, 738) concludes that the strength mandate is a barrier to intimate relationships and denies black women the companionship that they need. Barbara, a black woman of low SES, elaborates on the silencing of infertility:

BARBARA: I wouldn't say [I know] a lot [of people with infertility] because there—I—I bet it's not something you just readily talk about with people. I guess I have my one girlfriend, I talk about it with her because she's my friend and I know her history and she knows mine. But other than that, no . . . not really. . . . It's not something you talk about. . . . I think it's probably not as open a subject for discussion in my community as it would be in some others.

ANN: ... And why do you think that is?

BARBARA: I think it's just cultural differences. And that's the only thing I can attribute—attribute it to is just cultural differences. And it's just sort of the things you don't discuss ... that just is. And I don't know that it's necessarily any different than it would be for some other social—some other—some other groups either. I—I—I suspect that in some ways that other ethnic groups also would have the same kind of thing but just, you just don't do.

Keisha, a black woman of low SES, explains why she does not discuss her childbearing difficulties with others: "So I'm not going to tell [my mom] or nobody else because I know this is something I have to do because it's like personal (laughs) to me. So I wouldn't share it with nobody. But, you know, the person I'm going to be with or somebody like you (laughs). So yeah. That's like a tense situation for me.... And I can get on—on the computer all day and that's not going to help me. That's not going to do anything. Even if I told my mom, that's not going to do anything (laughs). So it's like—it's something I have to do." Keisha's motivation for being silent about her fertility struggles reflects the strength mandate imposed upon black women. To Keisha, infertility is a "personal" issue and "something she has to do" on her own to resolve. The belief that no one can help her but herself prevents her from sharing her struggles.

Ebony, a black woman of low SES, demonstrates the absence of infertility talk in her community: "I don't think I tell—do I tell people? (Pauses) I might have told two people but not really. The doctor and maybe—it's not that it's a secret. It's just that that's not really nothing that—I don't really find people that's really talking about it because most of my friends like I say have kids so where—I don't understand where that falls in the something to talk about, you know, for us." The silencing of infertility is so entrenched in Ebony's surroundings that she cannot even remember whether she discussed her issues with anyone. In addition to being an effect of cultural norms, the black women of low SES in this study did not talk about infertility because most of their peers have children. Troubles with childbearing are marginalized within social interactions, while childbearing itself is the center of conversation.

In addition to cultural practices, there are other reasons women of low SES, both black and white, do not discuss their fertility difficulties. For instance, by sharing their struggles the women are admitting that they want to become pregnant and are trying to conceive. This is problematic for some women of low SES because of the ideology that they should not be mothers in the first place. Despite the earlier childbearing norms, many of the participants of low SES reported having been criticized for being too young to attempt to have children. Roxanne, a black woman of low SES in her early twenties, states: "[I don't want to tell my mom] because she's—I don't know—she's going to say I'm too young. 'Why are you trying? You this. You that. You don't have a job right now. I'm too young to be a grandmother.' And that's the first thing she's going to say. And I'm looking at her like, 'You're almost fifty.' It's, 'I don't have any grey hair.' 'So?' I'm like, 'I don't care, Mom.' I'm like, 'When I'm ready, I'm going to be ready.'"

Julie, a white woman of low SES, has a similar experience: "Well, I wanted to talk to my mom about it but I never did. . . . And she asks but, you know, I—sometimes I lie to her and like, 'No, we're using protection,' you know, or whatever but, you know, I really—she thinks I should be further in my career to start having children but I think I've been working there a year and a half now and like I think I'm in there good enough." Julie and Roxanne are criticized by their mothers for wanting to have children; nevertheless, they aspire to the role, despite their young ages and lack of established careers. Julie and Roxanne negotiate with those stereotypes through avoidance or "information management" (Remennick 2000, 824); they either do not tell their mothers or choose to "lie" to them about their childbearing difficulties in order to avoid being criticized. Women of high SES do not face such conflict because they are viewed as embodying and fulfilling the norms of good motherhood, including the appropriate age to have a child.

Another explanation for low SES women's reluctance to talk about their fertility struggles was their fear of being embarrassed, stigmatized, or perceived as abnormal. The motherhood mandate makes motherhood seem natural among women, consequently making infertility, or the inability to achieve motherhood, seem unnatural. The women do not want to expose what they consider a weakness or an undesirable trait to others and choose not to disclose their childbearing problems (Miall 1986). Mikela, a black woman of low SES, explains:

ANN: Have you talked to many people about it?
MIKELA: Mm-mm.

ANN: No? Why?

MIKELA: 'Cuz, no! I'm not going to ruin that just—mm-mm.

ANN: What would you ruin?

MIKELA: Them knowing that I was abnormal for whatever reason, something wrong. Something else to talk about. Something that I don't need to be— that's none of their business. It's obviously up to me and God.

Mikela has not discussed her infertility with anyone because she is afraid that it will "ruin" her relationships due to its "abnormality." Her quote also reiterates the silence around personal issues in her community. She does not talk about it with others because "that's none of their business."

In addition to their embarrassment concerning infertility, some participants such as Ruby, a white woman of low SES, do not disclose their difficulties due to their inability to resolve them: "And that's something of that I think I hide most from people because I don't talk about my situation as much because I am more so embarrassed that I can't do something about it." Ruby is uninsured and therefore cannot access medical treatment for her infertility. The stereotype of infertility as a medical event is entrenched to the extent that Ruby is "embarrassed" by the fact that she cannot (medically) resolve her issues. In other words, she feels abnormal for her lack of access to medical treatment for infertility. This difference causes Ruby to refrain from discussing her childbearing difficulties with others. Ruby, however, turns to the Internet, which provides a safe virtual community in which she can discuss infertility without revealing her problems to others in her actual community: "I play an online video game once in a while and I have tons of friends on that. And I can tell one of my friends on there everything and anything and I feel good for the day and it's off my mind. You know, they aren't going to judge me past that. They aren't going to see me at the mall tomorrow doing the opposite of what I'm going to say, you know, sometimes. But I probably could not talk to someone else about it."

Ruby is able to discuss her fertility issues with her online "friends" because they do not "judge" her. The Internet's anonymity provides a safe haven for those with "concealable stigmatized identities" (McKenna and Bargh 1998, 683). She will not "see" them "tomorrow," which allows for anonymity and freedom of expression. The Internet forces a face-value conversation, one that is undisturbed by context, body language, and nonverbal cues. The anonymity allows users to escape the constraints of cultural taboos that forbid personal disclosure. Ruby can be herself without fear of repercussions or judgment.

Women of high SES are also hesitant to talk about their childbearing difficulties with others because of its stigma, but for different reasons. Jennifer, a white woman of high SES, explains:

ANN: Why don't you want people to know?

JENNIFER: I think it's because I'm embarrassed mostly.... Because it's not the natural order of things. Do you know what I mean?...I just—I don't know—I just—it's not right to me. Do you know what I mean? It's not—this isn't supposed to happen so. And I don't like people to feel sorry for me about anything.

Jennifer is "embarrassed" about her inability to conceive: it is "not the natural order of things." She has internalized the motherhood mandate and, as a result, feels abnormal and stigmatized. Rather than "ruin" relationships as in Mikela's case, Jennifer does not want others "feeling sorry" for her. This variation parallels the effects of infertility on partnerships: women of low SES feared men would leave them if they found out they were infertile, whereas women of high SES received support from their significant others.

Despite their hesitancy owing to the stigma associated with infertility, most women of high SES talked with others about their childbearing problems. Unlike Ebony, who attests to the taboo against discussing personal problems in the low SES black discourse, many women of high SES disclosed their fertility troubles precisely to quell conversation about them. Carole, a white woman of high SES, states: "Yeah, I [told] close friends and stuff. You do want some people to feel sorry for you and you do want people to shut up, too, like I say, you just have to tell 'em because you don't want them to ask you anymore (laughs). I'll—and I used to—I remember saying something like, 'You know, if there's any good news, I'll tell you. Don't, you know, don't keep asking me because it kills me and I die a little every time somebody asks me.' You do—you just die a little 'cuz, you know, they think they're just being cute and you're just like at your wit's end."

Ideologically, as a married, white, heterosexual woman of high SES in the United States, it is abnormal not to have children. Thus, a middle-class childless woman is likely to encounter questions. Carole told her close friends in an effort to "shut up" their constant inquiries about children.

"Coercive social exchanges" such as these in which women are forced to give information are commonplace in (high SES) experiences of infertility (Sandelowski and Jones 1986, 174). The pain of the questions was greater than the pain of revealing her difficulties. Because black women of low SES do not typically discuss this type of personal issue, such overt questioning was less common in their environments, although they nevertheless assumed that others disapproved of their childlessness.

Despite telling others about their struggles, most participants of high SES said their friends and family did not understand what they were going through. As Sarah, a white woman of high SES, explains: "I have several close friends and, you know, I don't know. They, you know, they say they understand but I know they don't. . . . And I do confide in a couple of close friends and I just feel like they're—they just feel really sorry for me. But no, they don't understand. They can't. My mother, she just—she's just sad. She can't understand it either. She says, 'I'll just listen but I don't know what to say.'" Sarah's friends "can't understand" what she is experiencing because they have not lived it, yet talking with others, such as her friends and mother, is a way Sarah copes with her infertility: "So yeah, I guess about two weeks ago [my husband] was like, 'I don't know. I think you need to go talk to somebody.' And I say, 'But I talk to everybody. This is my—that's my therapy,' you know, I talk to all of my friends and . . . it's like—I don't know . . . I don't know. Because I feel like—I guess I feel like I talk enough to people: to my friends and this friend at work and—I don't know." Disclosing her childbearing difficulties is Sarah's "therapy." She has maintained friendships and has supportive family members who are there to listen to her stories even if they cannot fully understand her experience.

Lindsey, a white woman of high SES who works at a local university, also talks with others as a way to deal with her fertility struggles: "And I think that's almost my—my outlet, you know, I really like to communicate with people and really pick their brains like, 'Oh, this happened to you? Well, what happened? You—or what did you do? You had another baby. Well, what worked for you?' You know? So really talking to other people about what worked and what didn't and just kind of hearing through the grapevine." For Lindsey, talking with others about her struggles not only provides her with emotional support, but she also discloses as a way to gain knowledge and resources about how to resolve her infertility, thereby reflecting and perpetuating the knowledge and resource gap between classes.

Infertility is a social experience that occurs outside the doctor's office or examining room: it takes place in the context of everyday lives. Race and class norms inform social practices, which in turn shape how women live with infertility. More specifically, reproductive, marital, and discursive norms shape women's social surroundings and how they live with infertility in such environments.

Peer groups and their reproductive practices differ by class, resulting in divergent infertility experiences. For women of low SES, as described by Ebony, "having kids is what they do"; therefore, it is difficult for the participants to relate to peers who "all" have children. For women of high SES, however, later childbearing norms cause more women to be childless. Additionally, accessibility to career and leisure opportunities allows the participants of high SES to relate to their peers, including those with children, about issues beyond mothering, and therefore allows them to maintain more friendships and receive more social support. It is easy to see how infertile women of low SES such as Ruby describe themselves as "oddballs." As economically marginalized women, they do not conform to the broader cultural stereotype of infertility. At the same time, their interpersonal relations are complicated because they do not fit in with their peers.

Marital norms, which vary by race and social class, also shape experiences of infertility. Culturally, black women of low SES marry less frequently and reject the notion that marriage is a prerequisite to having children. In turn, most participants of low SES in this study were unmarried. The impermanence of those relationships caused the women to fear that their partners would leave them upon learning of their childbearing difficulties. In contrast, to fulfill the life stages that place marriage before childbearing, all the women of high SES were married. Infertility tended to strengthen their relationships, and marriage was the strongest support system for the high-income women. In addition to marital support, the women of high SES were able to participate in infertility support groups and therapy, which remained beyond the reach of most women of low SES. Finally, discursive norms and taboos against discussing personal issues led black women of low SES to avoid talking about their infertility, yet disclosing their difficulties was a way the high-income women coped with their struggles and also furthered their support.

Examining the lived experience of infertility exposes the influence and impact of social norms on the condition. Such norms lead to wide variation in the experiences of high and low SES women. Infertility is not merely an objective experience that can be generalized to all women; rather, it is one based in ideological notions and influenced by the context in which it occurs. Indeed, how the women attempt to resolve their childbearing problems depends on the context in which they live. Infertility, then, is not merely a medical condition, but a quintessentially social phenomenon.

5

"Whatever Gets Me to the End Point"

••••••••••••••••••••

Resolving Infertility

I was thinking you could just get pregnant. I don't know what—well, [doctors] probably could tell me some stuff that I could do. But most doctors try to talk you out of getting pregnant.
—Michelle, black woman of low SES

I could tell that I knew more than [the doctor] did. I mean because I—I tend to do research and read anyway and I'm probably one of those patients who drive doctors crazy. . . . It wasn't until I got to my R.E. [reproductive endocrinologist] that I felt like she could answer my questions.
—Nadia, white woman of high SES

"Most doctors try to talk you out of getting pregnant," Michelle replied when I asked whether she had considered medical treatment for her infertility. For Michelle, a black woman of low SES, the negative comments she had come to expect from doctors made seeking infertility treatments simply unthinkable. In contrast, women of high SES, such as Nadia, could not imagine treating their infertility any other way; medical treatment was "*the* answer" to their childbearing difficulties. Such divergent experiences among women of different social classes resulted in dramatically different ways of resolving infertility.

Since the development of reproductive technologies in the 1970s and 1980s, infertility has increasingly been "medicalized," viewed as a disease and something to be treated rather than as a natural part of life (Bates and Bates 1996). Thus, one of the most common ways women attempt to resolve their infertility is through medical treatment. Accessing such treatment, however, is limited by a woman's class status, partly because medical institutions reflect what anthropologist Gay Becker (2000, 20) calls the "underlying moral economy of the U.S.," in part by limiting their services to select groups.

In the case of infertility, medical institutions serve as gatekeepers determining, according to stereotypes of good motherhood, who should and who should not mother. The medicalization of infertility lies at the intersection of mainstream ideas about medicine and motherhood. As I have argued, only certain groups are deemed worthy of motherhood (for example, white, affluent women), and medical institutions perpetuate that stereotype by providing the option of reproduction to some groups and withholding it from others. Medicaid covers contraceptive methods but not infertility treatments, while the reverse is true for several private insurers (King and Meyer 1997). Medical decision making reflects similar biases when physicians encourage affluent women to become pregnant but counsel poor women to use birth control (Fisher 1986). In other words, women are divided into "those for whom there is contraception if they'd only use it, and those for whom there are infertility treatments" (Cussins 1998, 73). Because of medicine's "cultural authority" and its aura of scientific objectivity, however, these processes often go unnoticed (Barker 2008, 29).

Health research also overlooks medicine's role in creating deep disparities in the treatment of infertility. Studies of inequalities in access to infertility treatment typically limit their analyses to financial barriers, such as its exorbitant cost and sparse insurance coverage, rather than considering social explanations for these disparities, such as discrimination, appointment scheduling, and doctor-patient relationships (for example, Henifin

1993; Staniec and Webb 2007). This narrow focus is particularly problematic because researchers have shown that even when insurance coverage is mandated and, in theory, all groups have access to infertility treatments, disparities persist. For instance, physicians Tarun Jain and Mark Hornstein (2005) found that in Massachusetts, a state with mandated comprehensive insurance coverage, the use of infertility services had indeed increased since implementation of the mandate, but it had done so among the same demographic group that receives treatment in other states without comprehensive insurance coverage—the white, wealthy, and educated; thus, the disparities remained. According to the authors, inequality was most significant along educational divides; of the patients receiving IVF services, none had less than a high school diploma, and 85 percent had attained at least a bachelor's degree from college. While subsequent researchers (Bitler and Schmidt 2012; Bitler and Schmidt 2006; Schmidt 2007) have echoed these findings, few, if any, studies have examined *why* the inequalities persist or what mechanisms (beyond obvious financial barriers) produce these inequalities (Bell 2010; White, McQuillan and Greil 2006).

Comparing the experiences of infertility among women of different socioeconomic groups allows us to explore the nuances of inequalities. I examine how medicine contributes to the development of disparities through its perpetuation of mainstream ideas about motherhood and reproduction. In other words, I explore the *social* exclusion of women of low SES from the ideals of motherhood and medicine (Bhalla and Lapeyre 1997). Examining the medical aspects of infertility reveals how women of low SES are marginalized along economic dimensions as well as social and political dimensions.

Attitudes toward Medical Solutions

Since the medicalization of infertility, medical treatment is assumed to be the best, if not the *only* solution for infertility. Therefore, all study participants pursue medical treatment or at least think about it in some form, but they do so in different ways. Women of low SES seek medicine, not for its treatment of infertility, but rather for an "answer" or diagnosis of why they are experiencing childbearing difficulties, whereas women of high SES pursue medicine for both diagnosis *and* treatment. Such differences are reflected in and may be attributed to the participants' attitudes about medical solutions to infertility as well as their structural and contextual circumstances.

How individuals make sense of health experiences varies according to their social location (Silva and Machado 2008). Research suggests that women of low SES, especially black women, are wary of medicine and many times do not seek medical treatment even when it is accessible. Black women dislike "external control of the body," as demonstrated by their rejection of breast-feeding (Blum 1999). Similarly, anthropologist Emily Martin (1990) found that working-class women tend to reject medical dominance over their bodies, particularly in relation to reproductive processes such as menstruation, while middle-class women internalize such views. Sociologist Sarah Franklin (1992) also suggests that women who are less concerned with adhering to dominant norms of reproduction, such as women of low SES in a culturally heterogeneous setting, are less likely to pursue IVF than are women of high SES who define their lives according to social conventions. Moreover, there is a historical mistrust of medicine among African Americans given the legacy of widely publicized abuses of medical power (Gamble 1997). Most notable among them are the infamous Tuskegee experiments, in which poor black men with syphilis were deliberately misled to believe they were receiving medical treatment, when in fact their disease was allowed to progress and remain untreated (Hill 1994).

These abuses cast a long shadow, producing a mistrust of hospitals and medical treatment, particularly a fear of medicines ingested into the body, such as pills and injections. For instance, black women are less likely to take oral contraceptives because of their beliefs that such birth control is a form of genocide (Thorburn and Bogart 2005). This belief is in part based on the long history of involuntary sterilizations of poor, black women and contraceptive policies that target poor women. Opinions of medical treatment for infertility also reflect how women approach reproduction more generally. As we learned in chapter 3, women of high SES use technological mechanisms to "try" to become pregnant, while women of low SES prefer more "natural" approaches.

In other words, black women do not merely reject medicine for its own sake. They are hesitant to accept and pursue medicine, particularly medical treatment ingested into the body, given its negative symbolic meaning developed from centuries of historical abuses. Such opinions and ideas are applied to resolving infertility (Molock 1999), as Barbara, a black woman of low SES, demonstrates when she told me, "I don't want to be somebody's science experiment." Veronica, a black woman of low SES, has similar sentiments regarding medical solutions for her infertility:

> VERONICA: The little injection things. I don't—I don't want to try that. I just want it to come, you know, naturally.
>
> ANN: Mm-hm. And what do you mean? What are the injections?
>
> VERONICA: I—I—I don't know what they're—that's what I said "the little injection" things. . . . And so I was like, "Yeah, I don't want that though." . . . And so I'm going to keep doing it the natural way. . . . Because I don't want to take no—because I—plus I don't know what that would do to me. You know, that might—I don't know what—I have been hearing horror stories about that and so I don't want any—yeah. . . . Like on the Internet. Like a baby might come out with a extra, you know, finger or a toe or—and I'm like, "Uh-uh." I don't want that to happen.
>
> ANN: How about reproductive technologies?
>
> VERONICA: No, mm-mm . . . I don't even want to—oh, that word is so nasty: repro—no, uh-uh. . . . I'm just—it makes me think of an alien baby or something. I don't—no. . . . That makes me—no, like a little green baby going to pop out or something . . . I don't want to look at them images. Just the word alone just— . . . It spooks me out.

Veronica is fearful about treating her childlessness medically, as she "doesn't know what that would do to [her]." Her understanding of medical resolutions stems from the Internet and "horror stories . . . about little injection things," which may also be rooted in black women's attitudes toward medicine more generally. Rachelle, a black woman of low SES, echoes Veronica's fears:

> RACHELLE: Like about a year and a half ago or two years [my doctor] had mentioned [treatments] to me and I told him I wasn't interested.
>
> ANN: Mm-hm. Explain to me in more detail why you're not interested in that.
>
> RACHELLE: I don't know. I just felt like—I don't know—kind of part of me felt like if it was meant for me to have 'em, I would have just had 'em. And—I don't know—I don't want to do anything that may harm me trying to have 'em when if it was meant to happen, I should have just had 'em.

Rachelle "is not interested" in treating her infertility medically because, like Veronica, she "feels like" having a child should come more "naturally." She is also concerned that the treatments may "harm" her and shatter her fatalistic hopes of having a child that is "meant" to be.

Low SES women's negative attitudes toward medically treating child-bearing difficulties stem from as well as contribute to their lack of familiarity with such treatments. Because the participants of low SES know few women in their social networks who are infertile, let alone use ARTs, most medical treatments for infertility are foreign and unfamiliar to them. Sherry, a white woman of low SES, "[doesn't] know anything" about reproductive technologies, and Angie, a black woman of low SES, does not "even know where to start to even think about" seeking medical treatment for her difficulties. Bonnie, a black woman of low SES, notes: "I'm sure there's a lot [of medical treatments] out there. I just don't know much about—I'd say probably the only thing I know about it is with the—the cleansing and in vitro cleansing stuff like that and then—I don't know—it was maybe about two months—I know it was this year where this—these two women, they went to a clinic and for some reason somehow they got pregnant and they were implanted with each other's eggs." Even though Bonnie works in a health care setting as a lab assistant, she "does not know much about" treating her childbearing issues medically. What knowledge she does have about infertility treatments derives from the media and reflects medical negligence.

Similar to their understanding of infertility and its stereotypes in general, most women of low SES receive their information about medical treatments for infertility through the media. Low SES women mention celebrities such as Angela Bassett, Sarah Jessica Parker, Celine Dion, and Connie Chung throughout their discussions of medical solutions for infertility. Tiffany, a single, black woman of low SES, states: "Like I have watched too many movies and like when people be going through that and needles and—and then like when it don't take and then when you do get pregnant, you end up pregnant with like six kids at once. I don't—I don't want that! That's too much. I just want one at a time or twins. I can do that. But as far as six-seven-eight kids in your stomach at one time, I know that's uncomfortable. . . . It was on like the Discovery channel, the Bio channel, or whatever there. That's just crazy." To Tiffany, the media presents medical treatments for infertility as "crazy" "needles" that result in multiple children. For those who are unfamiliar with medical treatment options and are part of a subculture in which medicine is not seen as trustworthy, the media becomes an outlet of information that perpetuates their fears.

Unlike women of low SES, remember that women of high SES "take charge of their fertility" through research and use of technology. Thus, when seeking information about resolving their childbearing difficulties, medical treatment is the preferred solution, and the women of high SES inform themselves about what it entails. Becca, a white woman of high SES, describes her interest:

ANN: So did you have a conversation with your husband before going to the fertility specialist . . . about seeking care and checking this out?

BECCA: Yeah, I think even before we got married I talked about it. . . . So I'm like, "Well, we'll give it six months. . . . You know, we'll try this. I'm doing everything I can think of and if it doesn't work, we'll go make, you know, an appointment."

Becca had a plan and timeline regarding her fertility. Before she even became aware of her difficulties she decided that she would resolve them medically and "make an appointment" with her physician should they arise.

Despite high SES women's overwhelming desire for medical treatment once childbearing problems began, they were still disappointed to learn that pregnancy required such intervention. Brooke, a nurse practitioner of high SES, reflects on her disappointment: "I am (pauses)—I am okay I think with the medications. And I can't decide how I feel about the technologies yet. Part of me just doesn't care. Whatever gets me to the end point. The end point is being pregnant and having a baby. That's fine. I'll do it. I don't care. I'll do it right now. You just tell me what I gotta do and I'll do it. And then part—another part of me really doesn't want to have to go there. Like I really—I don't want to have to go through some kind of, you know, very sterile, very impersonal treatment to have children." Brooke is open to resolving her childbearing difficulties medically because it will allow her to meet her "end point" or goal of having a child, but adhering to her life plan in such a manner is disappointing because it is not the typical way children are conceived. When she describes medical treatments as "sterile" or "impersonal," Brooke's comments evoke low SES participants' views of infertility treatments as "unnatural." She would prefer to have a baby with a partner rather than deliver one conceived in a test tube. Yet, like many other women of high SES, Brooke nevertheless believes that medicine is the answer to her difficulties, and she has high expectations for its success.

Colleen, a white woman of high SES, shares Brooke's optimism: "Oh, my gosh. This is the answer. An IUI [intrauterine insemination]. It's perfect. We're going to take, you know, we're going to make sure I have what I need and then we're going to make sure he has what he needs and we're going to put 'em together and of course it's going to be a baby. How could it not? How could you miss? It's perfect. And—and of course, you always know somebody who knows somebody who had that work the first time. And filled with all of that hope." For Colleen, medicine is the "answer" to her childbearing difficulties. The science behind it is "perfect" and "could not" fail. In contrast to women of low SES whose only references are to "horror stories" on television, Colleen's hopes are strengthened by knowing others whose infertility has been treated successfully. The high SES women's optimism and faith in medical technology is a direct contrast to low SES women's skepticism and mistrust of medicine.

"I Thought Maybe Only a Rich Person Could Do It": Inequalities in the Medical Treatment of Infertility

Infertility, as I have noted, is thoroughly medicalized: it is assumed to be a disease that requires a medical diagnosis and treatment. Thus, despite their very different attitudes toward medicine, women of both high and low SES who could not become pregnant ended up in the doctor's office. However, women of low SES who had childbearing difficulties went to the doctor in search of a diagnosis, while women of high SES wanted both a diagnosis *and* treatment of their childbearing difficulties. The differences in their reasons for seeking medical care reflect not only different attitudes toward medicine and reproductive technologies but also inequalities in the access and delivery of medical care in reproductive medicine.

Social psychologist Rosemary Davidson and her colleagues (2006) found that women of low SES are aware that their socioeconomic position contributes to the health disparities they face. Their "consciousness of . . . victimization" allows them to reflect upon the dominant society of which they are not a part as well as to develop ways to grapple with and resist the social forces that constrain them (Riessman 2000, 122). This recognition of inequality is rarely shared by individuals of high SES because privilege is often invisible. Indeed, women of low SES in this study are "outsiders-within" the medical context of infertility. They are marginalized by reproductive policies and practices, yet aware (albeit with limited knowledge) of the potential solutions they offer. This unique perspective gives them insight into the inequalities that are so much a part of reproductive medicine (Collins 1990). The following excerpt from my interview with Donna, a black woman of low SES, captures how economically disadvantaged women understand their own experiences of infertility through their awareness of higher-class women's experiences.

> No, I haven't [thought about medical options]. I haven't. My—it's probably a denial stage like I am more or less in denial but like I said, I see it on TV and you hear about it and it's like, "Wow, that sounds interesting." Let's see. Was it—I think it was Angela Bassett was the last thing I seen and she got twins but they took her egg out of her and put it in another woman and used her husband's sperm and I'm thinking, "Wow, that is quite a bit." So that was kind of amazing to me. But I know that's expensive so that's way like out of my league but that's something interesting and I thought about like, "Wow. She couldn't have kids and that was something really nice opportunity she had to have her own child so that was really nice." Yeah, but I haven't really looked like for myself . . .

Through media representations of infertility experiences, Donna is well aware of potential remedies, such as surrogacy, that are available for infertility, but she also acknowledges that those expensive solutions are "way out of [her] league" (Bell 2009). Donna's story reveals how the experiences of women of low SES deepen our understanding of infertility by reflecting upon both dominant *and* subordinate experiences and thus the powers that shape them.

The medical treatment of infertility is based on a "private medicalized market," in which "care is provided to consumers who can afford to pay for it, and other potential consumers are excluded" (Conrad and Leiter 2004, 161). This type of market results in a for-profit, business structure of the health care system (Bates and Bates 1996). As Carrie, a white woman of low SES, told me, "It's a money-making business is what it is." While fertility doctors may be "living the high life" according to Carrie, the institution of medicine cannot be reduced to such simplicity. The commercial activity is situated in and informed by a specific ideological context. In addition to securing a profit, medicine both reflects and perpetuates norms on which it is based. Consumers help drive the medical treatment of infertility, yet the institution of medicine still explicitly and implicitly determines who those consumers are based upon its foundation in social norms regarding who is and is not worthy of treatment.

As we learned in chapter 2, the middle- and upper-class ideals of motherhood are at odds with low SES women's lives. Similarly, the medical context of infertility, in which medicine is a "middle-class constituency," is incongruent with that of women of low SES (Steinberg 1997, 40). The sequence and scheduling of appointments is based on middle-class lifestyles, in which professional women have both autonomy and flexibility in their schedules at work and at home. Women of low SES who work, however, rarely have the power to determine their schedules. Nicole, a white woman of low SES originally from South Africa, laments:

The only way I could ever talk to [physicians] is if I have an appointment and I don't understand that. And they—it's like they don't understand that, you know, we can't just always pay $20 all the time or $25 every time just to have an appointment just to talk to you for two seconds. You know, and that's the frustrating part is that they don't get it. And then they always want you to have an appointment in the middle of the day and, you know, well, you know, I go to work to be able to afford this appointment (laughs), you know? It's—and it's very frustrating. Yeah, so I mean like last year I went to doctors' appointments so many times and it was—I had to work, you know, my bosses were giving—giving me like, "Okay, why do you have so many doctors' appointments?" And, "I'm, you know, dealing with a lot of stuff and medical issues right now" and luckily I kept my job, you know, they didn't let me go or anything, which I was really grateful for and so everybody understood and this year I just let it go for the most part because I just can't do that all the time. Just—I mean my job is my number-one priority right now. I've got to keep my job.

The appointment structure of reproductive care is an example of how medicine is organized around the interests of patients of high SES and neglects the circumstances of low SES women's lives. This is particularly true of infertility practices, which cater to affluent women who can afford to pay for treatment out-of-pocket. Nicole had to "let [fertility treatment] go" because of the inflexibility of her job. In a sense, she had to choose between having a family and earning a living, a choice many women of higher economic standing do not confront. Physicians, however, "don't get" the dilemma in which they have placed Nicole because they view their patients' schedules through a middle- and upper-class lens and are unaware of the patients' social contexts.

Health care's failure to understand the lived experience of infertility outside the doctor's office may explain why even when women are insured, as in states with comprehensive coverage, disparities still exist. For instance, according to some participants, physicians conduct more procedures when they are aware a patient is insured in order to get maximally reimbursed. This excessive use of procedures is especially troublesome for women with limited disposable income, for whom the extra fees and more frequent co-pays constitute significant expenses. Jackie, a white woman of low SES, describes this difficulty: "I mean because I have insurance, [physicians] try to put me on this stuff, which I understand because our health coverage is great. All we've had to pay through this thing is like $40 to the doctor's office. . . . But our actual prescription insurance is really awful and they put me on Premicare 1, which is the prenatal vitamins so they told me. And it was like a $92 co-pay every month I have to pay. . . . And I mean we have a very tight budget because I don't work and that $92, I mean it doesn't really fit in (laughs)." Taking prenatal vitamins "doesn't really fit in" to Jackie's budget. She is forced to prioritize and navigate all the services offered. Physicians' lack of awareness of their patients' financial circumstances, coupled with the incentives to order more tests and do more procedures in a fee-for-service system, causes them to overlook excessive expenses. In effect, insurance places more constraints on those less financially well-off and hinders the proper care of women of low SES. Even when treatments are accessible, a hierarchy of care remains.

In addition to disparities caused by the presence or absence of insurance, the *type* of insurance shapes physicians' responses to infertility treatment.

Keisha, a black woman of low SES, describes her denial of medical care based on her status as a Medicaid recipient:

ANN: So have you ever talked to [the doctor] about becoming pregnant besides, you know, when you go in for [other reasons] . . . ?

KEISHA: No, because I feel they're going to be like, you know, you're on Medicaid and you—they don't cover for this and that and this and that. And I don't want to be let down like that, you know, I really don't. And I feel because I'm on Medicaid, I do try to get some help in some other way and that—and they're like, "Well, you're on Medicaid, you know, you shouldn't be, you know, trying to do all of this on Medicaid."

Medicaid does not cover infertility treatments. In addition to this explicit exclusion, however, Keisha is implicitly excluded from receiving fertility care because of her fear of being "let down." She has been told too often that she should not be "trying to do all of [these things] on Medicaid" so she avoids that conversation altogether by not inquiring about her infertility. Medicaid is a status marker for class. Not only does this preclude the inclusion of infertility treatment coverage within its policy, but it also shapes the treatment women on Medicaid receive from physicians. A three-tiered system shapes access to infertility treatments: elective treatments for those who can afford to pay out-of-pocket, private insurance for those who are covered, and public insurance for the poor—to say nothing of the forty million Americans who have no insurance at all. Thus, such policies, by making infertility treatments accessible to the affluent and beyond the reach of the poor, have historically regulated who can and should reproduce and mother (Steinberg 1997).

The circumstances surrounding the doctor-patient relationship further perpetuate the exclusion of women of low SES from receiving medical care for their infertility. Physicians, considered experts, are revered as authorities about all health-related things (Freidson 1972). Sociologist Sue Fisher (1986) has argued that women, particularly marginalized women, have been socialized to accept the authority of others. Tamara, a black woman of low SES, demonstrates such submission when she told me that she "just let [the doctor] do her job and felt like it was going to be right." Such a reluctance to assert themselves with physicians leads some women of low SES not to mention their childbearing difficulties because they assume the doctor will identify problems if they exist. Donna, a black woman of low SES, is one such example:

> Yeah, but still if they tell me everything normal, then that kind of ease for me instead of me telling them like, "Oh, I can't have a baby. Could you tell me"— I'm thinking if they check me up and then they'll let me know if they find something wrong. So that's my way of thinking of it. And probably me not wanting to hear it (laughs). They do—yeah, me putting them onto, "Well, oh, take this test. And this is what's wrong with you." So yeah. Every time I go like give blood work and everything but that's normal and so that kind of soothes me like, "Mm, maybe nothing is wrong." So yeah.

Donna is reassured that "everything [is] normal" when the doctor does not indicate otherwise. She waits for the physician to identify or probe about an issue rather than introducing it herself. The doctor, not Donna herself, is the expert about Donna's body. Donna's experience reflects the highly asymmetrical nature of the medical interview, which discourages many patients from bringing up their concerns. Physicians typically maintain tight control over the structure of the interview; they ask the questions and manage the progression of topics. These asymmetries are heightened when barriers of race, class, and gender separate doctors from their patients (Willems et al. 2005).

The communication (and contextual) divide between the highly educated doctors and the less educated women pursuing care caused many of the women of low SES to discontinue medical treatment for their infertility. Jocelyn, a black woman of low SES, reflects upon such interaction:

> ANN: Did they explain to you why you needed [infertility treatment]?
> JOCELYN: Not really. They just, you know, they didn't—they didn't even give me a booklet. I had to find me a book and research on my own. [How can you] be a physician and [get] a degree and . . . not [be] open with the patients and you're not showing them that you're caring? . . . I had to do everything by myself. I had to buy a $25 book; [money] that I could have . . . kept in my pocket . . .
> ANN: Because the doctors wouldn't explain it to you?
> JOCELYN: Not like they did—I mean just they come back, "Take these pills, you know, for three months. Come back." (laughs) I mean that's crazy.

In this brief dialogue, Jocelyn highlights numerous ways in which her inter-action with her physician was negative and unproductive. The doctor failed to explain to Jocelyn either the nature of her reproductive problem or the purpose of the medication. Jocelyn experienced this doctor's poor communi-cation as evidence of an uncaring attitude.

Jocelyn's experience is not unique. Researchers have found that the failure to inform patients about the purpose of medication is commonplace (Tarn et al. 2006) and that physicians give more information to educated patients (Anspach 1993). In the case of Jocelyn, this was the only medical treatment she received for her infertility. The lack of communication and its negative tone led her to seek out her own sources of information and not to return for follow-up care. Similarly, Bonnie, a black woman of low SES in her early thir-ties, did not pursue the physician's prescribed treatment because it was "too complicated" to fit into her life:

> Oh, he gave me some pills. He gave me some pills to take. I'm like, "Oh, I'm tired of taking pills."... I didn't take 'em.... Like it was—it was weird because I was supposed to take this like the first three days and then take something the next five days. I'm thinking, "Look, this is too much. Sometimes I don't even know what two-plus-two is." You know? So what makes you think I'm going to remember to do that? I mean he had got a calendar out and drew it out and this and that and then. And my fiancé's supposed to go to some kind of clinic and give his sperm and I'm like, "Uh-uh, no"... that's too complicated.

While the physician was trying to be helpful, he did not realize the regimen of infertility treatment was too complex for Bonnie's circumstances. By not simplifying the treatment or assisting Bonnie in better understanding how she may adapt her circumstances to adhere to the treatment, Bonnie was left without any solution.

Miscommunication and health literacy and its effects are further demon-strated in the experience of Kayla, a shy, black woman of low SES:

> ANN: Did you ever go to the doctor to ask about it?
> KAYLA: No. I always tried to ask them do they have something to help me get pregnant but they say no.
> ANN: Do you—do you know of anything that they could have done for you?

KAYLA: No, but my brother's baby mama told me that they had some type of pills that can help you get pregnant because she heard it from her auntie but she don't remember what the pills was called. And she told me to ask them but they said no.

Kayla lacks knowledge about the specific treatments available for infertility. Instead of telling the doctors about her difficulties conceiving, perhaps due to the practice of not disclosing personal issues, Kayla inquires about "something to help [her] get pregnant." Given this phrasing, the physicians may not have understood Kayla's troubles. This misunderstanding coupled with the stereotype that young, poor, black women are bad mothers, may have led the doctors to say "no" to Kayla's request.

Many times doctors rely on their authority as experts to discourage unfit mothers from reproducing. "Doctor knows best," the watchword of physicians' institutional authority, is exemplified in their interactions with patients. Doctors advise patients and many times attempt to persuade them by "implying dire consequences" if the patient does not comply (Fisher 1986, 4). This tactic is evident in Keisha's experience. She describes an interaction with physicians after she had a miscarriage at age sixteen: "They—they just—they just seem like they just didn't want me to have any kids (laughs) at all. At all. And that was sad. They, you know, they scared me into even trying to have any more. They tried—they tried to get me not to even have anymore. . . . They was really scaring me. That's why I—I said, 'Oh (laughs). Never again, Holy Grace Hospital. Never again.' Because they scared me and it was just—just crazy."

Although physicians "scared" Keisha into not trying to have any more children, she subsequently had two children and is now suffering from secondary infertility, or the inability to become pregnant or to carry a pregnancy to term following the birth of one or more biological children. Yet the incident Keisha describes, occurring nearly two decades ago, has prevented her from seeking medical care for her current childbearing difficulties. "Never again" will Keisha seek the care of medical professionals regarding her trouble conceiving, which in turn serves to further drive the class-based divide of medical treatment for infertility.

Josie's experience also exposes the doctor-patient relationship as one based in power:

So I was actually thinking about going to see someone else . . . And I'm just like, "Do I really want to start over with someone else?" And then at the same time I don't want to like hurt his feelings—not like hurt his feelings but like, you know, I don't want to—I don't want him to feel like I am stepping over him to get a second opinion but I kind of am because you're not really, you know, telling me anything. So I'm not for sure if I'm going to see this other doctor or not. I've been thinking about it. I guess I'm still thinking about it as to what I'm going to do with that.

Josie, a black woman of low SES, is dissatisfied with her current practitioner because he "isn't telling [her] anything." Yet, despite this dissatisfaction, she is hesitant to switch providers for fear that she will be "stepping over him" and "hurt his feelings." To Josie, there is a clear hierarchy of care that she is fearful to disrupt. In turn, she sacrifices the quality of the care she receives for her childbearing issues.

The influence of doctor-patient communication on the experience and construction of infertility is also apparent among women who did not receive medical care *specifically* for their infertility issues. Given their marginalized status and construction as bad mothers, many participants of low SES perceived discrimination from medical providers when they requested reproductive health care during general medical visits. These experiences can deter the women from seeking such care. Psychologists Mary Breheny and Christine Stephens (2007) found in their research on teen mothers that the young women avoided medical care because of the negative reactions they received from health professionals. The authors conclude that the "wider discursive context of 'judgmental' health care provision" must be taken into account when examining the utilization of medical care among marginalized populations (Breheny and Stephens 2007, 123). Such a context is evident in the reproductive health care experience of Michelle, a black woman of low SES in her mid-twenties:

ANN: Have you been to the doctor about [your infertility]?

MICHELLE: No . . . because I thought that, I was thinking you could just get pregnant. I don't know what—well they probably could tell me some stuff that I could do. But most doctors try to talk you out of getting pregnant.

Michelle could not conceive of seeking medical help for infertility given her previous interactions with physicians in which they tried to "talk

[her] out of getting pregnant." Michelle's negative experiences with doctors excluded her from reproductive medicine in two ways: first, by discouraging her from even trying to become pregnant, and second, by causing Michelle to *anticipate* that she would continue to experience similar treatment, which subsequently prevented her from seeking medical assistance when she was having difficulty conceiving. They discouraged both her fertility as well as the resolution of her infertility.

Tiffany, a black woman of low SES, attributes such discrimination to being African American:

> Like if like most—like if [my friends and I] wanted to go in there to get tested and stuff like that, [the doctor] always like trying to push you to get like the little UID [IUD] or whatever. . . . And like we like, "We don't want to be on birth control. Why are you trying to make us get on this?" And then like she'll just give us condoms and stuff. Okay, that's fine and dandy but you don't have to just like always push it at us, you know, as black people or— . . . I don't know. She was just really rude. I think that's another reason why I really didn't get no help because she was my doctor there. . . . It was—it was plenty of us that she did that to. Like she used to try to force us to take birth control. And like she was like, "You should try this. You should do this. You should do that." I am not going to do it because I don't want to . . . I don't want to be on the pill. I don't want to—be on the patch. I don't want the shot and I don't want that UID thing. Y'all are not sticking that in me. . . . I'm like, "I'm trying to get pregnant. Not trying not to get pregnant."

Tiffany was limited to seeking care at a low-income health clinic, which had only one doctor. This structural barrier intersected with ideological barriers because this particular physician, according to Tiffany, employed racial stereotypes by discouraging rather than encouraging her reproduction so Tiffany "really didn't get . . . help" for her infertility.

Some women of low SES reported discrimination along demographic characteristics beyond race, including marital status. According to the norms and conventions of high SES culture, which is also the culture of physicians, only married individuals should have children. Thus, as in the case of Lisa, a white woman of low SES, physicians discouraged unmarried women from becoming pregnant:

I did have one doctor that she just wanted to do a hysterectomy and get it over with. . . . And I was—it was when I was thirty-two. She was like, "Well, you're thirty-two and not married. Do you really want to have kids?" I'm like, "What does it have to do with being married to anyone?" You know. And, you know, when I—I was dating the guy in Cleveland and she's like—"How do you expect to get pregnant when you don't live together?" And I'm like, "I know lots of people who get pregnant and don't cohabitate. This isn't—they're not directly related to each other."

Lisa's unmarried status led her physician to suggest a hysterectomy rather than considering other options to resolve Lisa's reproductive problems. This encounter illustrates the clash of norms between a patient, who belonged to a culture that accepted single parenthood, and her doctor, whose culture disapproved of single parenthood.

Ultimately, the women's experiences of exclusion from medical treatment for infertility become seemingly normal, thereby reinforcing the stereotype that infertility occurs among economically and racially dominant groups. Because of this, many women of low SES in the study consciously or unconsciously accept mainstream notions of classed infertility, failing to recognize the forces behind such inequality. The stereotype of infertility as a higher-class issue, perpetuated in medicine, meant that Candace, a black woman of low SES, did not even try to seek treatment. She told me, "I believe I could have did a lot of things to change it. I didn't think—I didn't think—I thought maybe only a rich person could do it maybe. Or maybe—I don't know—maybe—I didn't think I could really do it like get a—get fertility pills or get my uterus scraped or—I had heard of things but maybe I didn't really think I could do it." Candace interpreted the medical treatment of infertility as something for the "rich." The exclusion of women of low SES from medicine was normalized in that Candace cannot articulate why only a "rich person could do" infertility treatments. In turn, she perpetuates such understandings and thus her exclusion by not pursuing medical care for her infertility.

Sharply contrasting with the experiences the women of low SES described, were those of the women of high SES who sought medical treatment to resolve their childlessness. Not only are women of high SES financially able to afford infertility treatments, but they are also included, both structurally and ideologically, in mainstream medicine. Their stories suggest that they believe they are in control of their treatment and in partnership with physicians for their reproductive care.

The middle-class bias apparent in medical institutions conforms to the needs, schedules, and resources of women in that same class location. Unlike women of low SES, women of high SES are able to attend the frequent appointments required for infertility treatment because their work schedules are flexible or because their partners' incomes are high enough to allow them not to work. Sarah, a white woman of high SES, describes her ability to adapt to medicine's rigid requirements: "[My supervisor] came into my office and she's been so supportive all along and she said something like, 'You've been asking for too much time off to go to doctor's appointments. You know, you need to be able to change these. You need to be—to pay attention to your schedule' and whatever. . . . But she retracted her statement to once I started crying and—and telling her, 'You can't go on any other day or any other time.'" Like Nicole, Sarah had difficulty juggling all of the appointments required by infertility treatments, but, unlike Nicole, Sarah had the status and agency to be able to negotiate with her supervisor to continue medical care. Being able to talk back to one's superior—and to prevail—is a privilege not all women enjoy.

This privilege also extends to interactions with physicians. For women of high SES, the doctor-patient relationship was more of a partnership than one based in power differences. Similar demographic characteristics placed the women of high SES on a more equal plane with physicians. Additionally, the increased agency and control typical among women of high socioeconomic settings also diminished the hierarchy of care that was so prominent in low SES women's experiences. They are accustomed to "taking charge" of their reproduction (Lareau 2003).

The casual equality apparent in high SES women's relationships to their physicians is exemplified by Colleen, a white woman of high SES, who called her physician, "Brian," by his first name. They were friends, peers, and equals, working together to resolve her childbearing difficulties. This scenario significantly contrasts with the authority and distance women of low SES ascribe to their physicians, which ultimately affects their care. In other words, unlike women of low SES, women of high SES are so immersed in the medical experience that their inclusion becomes a normal part of their daily routines. Nadia, a white woman of high SES, describes her interaction with physicians:

I could tell that I knew more than [the doctor] did. I mean because I—I tend to do research and read anyway and I'm probably one of those patients who drive doctors crazy but it's not like I'm going on like chat rooms or, you know, random web forums. I'm really doing research and I still had access to the online medical library from when I was doing my MBA so I would access medical trials and read and I just didn't feel like she knew much. It wasn't until I got to my R.E. [reproductive endocrinologist] that I felt like she could answer my questions. . . . I lied actually. I had only been trying for six months but I told her I had been trying a year because I had a feeling that it was going to be problematic and I didn't want to waste any more time.

Rather than being discouraged from getting pregnant like Michelle, Nadia actually went to physicians with her own diagnoses, questions, and treatment ideas. Her access to resources and knowledge allowed Nadia to believe that she "knew more" than the first physician she visited. Additionally, in contrast to the women of low SES who were excluded from the system, Nadia had the agency and ability to know how to work the system. Because she knew the medical definition of infertility, she was able to exaggerate the length of time she had been trying to get pregnant, a tactic that allowed her to gain access to infertility treatments earlier in addition to winning the respect of her reproductive endocrinologist (R.E.). Unlike Tamara who "let the doctor do her job," Nadia was in control of the medical interaction.

Such active presence in the high SES women's medical care is further demonstrated by Becca, a white woman of high SES, who explains:

I was like on the accelerated plan. I found out every single test I had to have, figured out where in my cycle it had to be done and got everything done in like two months. . . . But I mean like that CDC website I went through every single clinic and then made a spreadsheet for my age range. And then when I would go into the doctor's office, I had all of the tests and they were all color coded with little tabs and like a little notebook. I do, you know, looking back like most people throw like a manila envelope at 'em, you know, with their tests in 'em and they're like, "Did you want this back?" And I'm like, "No, that's your copy."

Rather than wait the one year to seek infertility treatment, as indicated by the medical definition of infertility, Becca was "on the accelerated plan."

She not only had the ability but also the knowledge to dictate her own timeline of care. Unlike Donna who depended on the physician to tell her if something was wrong, Becca took information to the doctors rather than wait to receive it from them. Becca researched which fertility specialists were the most successful for her age group, and in her words, "interviewed them" for the best fit. In contrast to the experiences of women of low SES who were limited by their insurance or low-income status to certain doctors and clinics, such as Tiffany, Becca "did [her] homework" and had the privilege of choice when selecting a care provider.

Whereas women of low SES, such as Josie, were fearful of "stepping over" their physicians to switch doctors, women of high SES frequently made such transitions. Stephanie, a white woman of high SES, elaborates: "[The doctor was] like, 'Oh, you just haven't given it enough time' basically. And I thought, 'Well, I think I have' after, you know, at this point I'm thinking, 'I have. I've given it a lot of time in my book.' And—and so I waited for a few more months and then I went, 'You know, I'm still not happy with that answer and I feel not valued. I feel like my—my voice still needs to be heard. Like there's got to be something more.' So I got a recommendation from somebody else and saw another doctor. . . . And for the first time I felt like validated." It was important to Stephanie that "her voice be heard," as she is used to such acknowledgment in her daily life. She disagreed with the physician on the timing of infertility treatment, which diminished her confidence in the physician's expertise (or technical knowledge) and went elsewhere. Stephanie had the support and resources to get a recommendation for a different physician, which allowed her desires and ideas to be "validated."

Such teamwork and equality inherent in the high SES women's discussions of their medical interactions is exemplified in the experience of Iris, a white woman of high SES, who told me: "[After receiving the infertile diagnosis] we just tried—we suddenly went into like, 'What can we do— what anything we can do. What can we do?' And it seemed—it—it was like, 'Well, you just wash [the sperm].' We'll just, you know, we just went in there like to the clinics saying like, 'Just wash 'em. That should work.'" Iris and her husband had an active response that placed them on the same level as the physician. "What can *we* do," as if a team, was their initial reaction to her husband's diagnosis of infertility. The presumed ease of overcoming their reproductive problems, implied by their suggestion to simply "wash" the sperm, indicates their presumed ability to overcome most difficulties they have faced in life. In their minds and in their context, Iris and her husband should be able to control their infertility, including its resolution.

Not only are women of high SES structurally included in the medical treatment of infertility, but their inclusion also goes unrecognized as it reflects their own circumstances in which they typically have control and access to their desires and equality (if not superiority) in their relationships. Women of high SES have the ability to choose their physician, how and when their care will take place, and what that care will entail. They are socialized to have the tools to intervene in medical institutions and get what they want (Lareau 2003). For women of high SES, doctors are neither the experts nor the gatekeepers who determine what information is given and received; they provide a means to an end in which the higher-class women themselves dictate their care plans. In other words, unlike women of low SES who are excluded from receiving medical care for their infertility, women of high SES have the option of excluding certain doctors from treating them for their childbearing difficulties.

In reproductive medicine, the organization of medical practice supports this partnership. Because some infertility treatments, such as IVF, are not covered by insurance in most states, patients who undergo these treatments must be able to afford to pay for them out-of-pocket. Patients who pay for their own treatments can exercise significant leverage in the doctor-patient relationship. Thus, medical practices treating infertility are at least partly client-dependent or dependent for their financial survival on patients, who refer themselves directly (Freidson 1960). Physicians in infertility practices are typically accustomed to dealing with affluent patients who expect to be treated collegially—patients who in other settings might be seen as demanding.

Beyond Medicine: Other Options to Resolve Childlessness

Medicine is not the only option for resolving infertility. Indeed, many participants were begrudgingly confronted with the "why-not-just-adopt" inquiry from friends and family, but adopting a child is not such a simple solution. Like medicine, adoption is situated in a social context. Stereotypes shape its practices and policies, including the definition of a good parent and who can have access to adoption services. According to reproduction scholar Charis Thompson (2005), adoption is a form of social engineering in which its home study or parental screening system is informed by race, class, sexuality, and marital stereotypes, all of which result in exclusionary practices to create an ideal family. Social class permeates all levels of the adoption process (Rothman 1989). The women relinquishing their children for adoption are typically of a lower SES than those seeking to obtain children through adoption. Open adoption has become a type of commodified motherhood through which children are "bought" and "sold," a system that advantages those with higher incomes. In some states, such as California, in which private, open adoption is the norm, prospective parents create brochures—advertisements for the happy homes they will provide—and market themselves directly to birth mothers. The entire process is brokered by private attorneys. Needless to say, birth mothers are likely to choose affluent, two-parent homes to provide all the advantages to their babies. In other words, in this market, "adoption is as much a class issue as it is anything else" (Rothman 1989, 130). Additionally, private or church-affiliated adoption agencies typically have other exclusionary policies, such as age limits or requirements that prospective parents be married.

Aware of their exclusion from medical options for resolving infertility, the women of low SES in the study also acknowledge their marginalization by adoption policies. Judy, a white woman of low SES, states that: "I have thought about [adoption] but then I don't think that—I don't think they would give me a baby because I'm not married and, you know, they don't just give any old person a baby. Especially when you don't have like a lot of money and, you know?" Judy is open to adopting a child, yet she recognizes that her social class and marital status will make adoption unlikely. Because "they don't just give any old person a baby," Judy has not pursued adoption.

In addition to implicitly excluding poor and working-class women from adoption by judging parental adequacy at least partly on monetary criteria, adoption is explicitly prohibitive for women of low SES because of its financial cost. Jessica, a white woman of low SES in her late thirties, explains:

[The cost is prohibitive], mm-hm, yeah. We just weren't and still aren't, you know, even when we looked at adoption. You know, 'cuz we seriously talked about adoption after a while. . . . You know, which is still again, you know,

$20,000. $15–$20,000. I'm like—and it's all cash up front. I'm like, "We don't have, you know." I'm like, "I'm working full-time and going to school just to pay the house payment and everything else 'cuz, you know, my husband's laid off every other month or six months from the automotive industry." You know, and now he's going back to school and so forth. But I'm like, "I don't ever see us just having, you know, $15–$20,000 cash to do." So it's like, you know, we never give up on the idea. It's like and I guess somewhere in the back of my head I never give up on, you know, it's like, "Well, maybe that miracle will still happen." I don't hold my breath anymore but I think there's a part of you that just can't ever let go of that hope that, you know.

As a working-class woman, Jessica is unable to make the "up front" costs required for adoption. Her husband's insecure job, along with their educational costs, does not leave room for extra expenses. Being able to adopt would be a "miracle" for Jessica, but she is "not holding her breath."

For the majority of women of high SES, including those who adopted, adoption was their second choice after medical treatments, a view that in part reflects the medicalization of infertility, which has made medicine the favored resolution and further perpetuates biological motherhood as the norm (Franklin 2013). The secondary status of adoption is also due to the "motherhood mandate" in which women are expected to bear children naturally (Letherby 2002; Russo 1976). Nadia, a white woman of high SES, clearly articulates this view:

Sometimes I don't even like to think about [adoption] because then that means there's no hope for my own biological kids. And in some ways, it's like it's very egoic. I recognize that because if you want kids, what difference does it make if they're your own? Well, okay, fine, let's say you even get past that. So the thing is people are like, "Well—" and I—I really want to strangle people who say, "Well, you can always adopt." As if that's easy. Well, on average it's about $30,000 to adopt a newborn. It takes several years. It takes a lot of—you will go through so much scrutiny that—to get—go through the approval process to be adoptive parents. . . . It's like any idiot off the street can have kids but to adopt, you have your life torn apart. You have to have interviews for everything. Everything tested. All kinds of stuff. They come through your house. They look at everything. You know, you have to perf—you know, basically you're on, you know, you have to perform perfectly. You have to prove that you're worthy to be a parent as if you haven't gone through enough proving in your own mind and feeling of unworthy. . . . In fact, we're starting on the process just because I don't want to reach the end of the biological road and find, "I have to do another two years worth of stuff leading up to that." So just in our back pocket. So yeah, I'm not thrilled about it. But I figure, "If it gets to that point, I will be happy." But I don't think the—the adoption process is very great here either.

The social construction of parenthood, family, and mothering has developed a hierarchical distinction between biological motherhood and social motherhood (Letherby 1999). This "blood bias," or preoccupation with biological kinship, is central to our cultural understanding of family (Franklin 2013; Parry 2005b, 276). Such thinking is reflected in Nadia's opposition to adoption because it means "there is no hope for [her] own biological kids." Adoption is her "back pocket" option that she will force herself to be "happy" about should it come down to that. Like the women of low SES, Nadia recognizes the complexity and scrutiny involved in the adoption process; yet, unlike women of low SES, Nadia is able to afford it and has the race, class, and marital characteristics of a good parent. She is not fearful of her exclusion from adoption; she is fearful of having it become her only option (Miall 1989).

In addition to privileging biological motherhood over social motherhood, many women of high SES are hesitant to adopt because it diminishes the amount of control they have over the childbearing process. Sarah, a white woman of high SES, elaborates:

> I guess the biggest thing is we're very conscious over food and what we put into our bodies, my husband and I. And so it's like if I don't know exactly where this child has come from and like—I don't know—that's the piece. It's like this whole—it's the—it's the nature part that—I don't know—I don't know if I could deal with someone else's and not knowing what was going to surface as the years go on. I think that's the piece that I'm like, "Really?" But I think—I don't know if I could ever let that go. I don't know. Like, "Will this kid end up with something?" It's like at least I can—I feel like I guess when I am pregnant, I can control what I do and what the unborn fetus is getting or not getting.

Sarah and her husband are afraid to adopt because they are not in "control" of the birth family's genes or of the birth mother's health behavior during pregnancy—both of which they see as a source of problems that can surface later. Sarah and her husband know their bodies, their history, and how they care for themselves, but they do not have that knowledge about others' lives. Being in control is an important part of Sarah's life, and she fears that the ultimate outcome of the adoption will be shaped by forces she cannot control.

Despite their hesitancy and negative views about adoption, five out of the fifty-eight participants ultimately resolved their childlessness by adopting a child. Three of those five participants were middle class, and two were working class who received the money for adoption as gifts from friends and family. The higher prevalence of adoption among middle-class women may be reflective of the ability of wealthy, upper-class women to pursue medical treatments longer and the low SES women's economically and socially unfavorable position in the "adoption market." Like medical infertility treatment, adoption is expensive so, for middle-class women on fixed incomes, the "odds" of success become a factor in decision making. Adoption promises a much greater likelihood of having a child at the end of the process than does a single round of IVF, yet they are approximately equivalent in cost. Stephanie, a white, middle-class woman, with an annual household income of approximately $55,000, explains such reasoning:

> [The doctor] said, "Well, here's a couple options for you. But if you're interested in not going any further with the process of, you know, to blowing out your tubes" and like all of these different things that she talked to us about, "then I really think that if you are—if you are longing so desperately to still be parents, that maybe adoption is the way for you all to go." . . . And she said, "I can pretty much guarantee that if you go adoption route, there may be bumps in ro—and bruises but you're not going to have the—the chance of disappointment in the extreme sense that you would if—if we go down this [medical] path because you still may not conceive, depending on what we find."

After several infertility tests and a few drug treatments, Stephanie and her husband were faced with surgeries as the remaining medical options to resolve their infertility. Due to their financial concerns over such procedures, their physician suggested they consider adoption because it is more of a "guarantee" of a child compared to the "extreme disappointment" that may ensue with continuing medical care. They heeded the physician's advice and adopted twin boys "who were born in [their] hearts."

While not permanent, foster care is another solution to overcoming involuntary childlessness. None of the women of high SES were open to becoming foster parents, yet several of the participants of low SES not only liked the idea, but they actually preferred it to biological motherhood. The openness to foster care among the women of low SES reflects their familiarity with foster care in their lived environments. Most women of low SES know of others, if not themselves, who were fostered as children. Jodi, a white woman of low SES, is such an example: "Yeah, there—there is adoption and, you know, if—if I did find out later in life that I really can't have children then, you know, I would think about fostering or adopting because I, you know, that's what happened with me. I—I was given that chance. So, you know, why not give it to somebody else who needs it? And you already know what, you know, you have been through so you know what to do and what not to do and what signs to look for if you get a hel-lion (both laugh)." Jodi was "given a chance" through foster care as a child so she is open to the idea of becoming a foster parent. Her past experiences give her knowledge and confidence in her own ability to foster; among women of high SES these components are missing, which prevents them from pursuing this social mothering option.

Like Jodi, Regina, a quiet and reserved black woman of low SES, also wants to be a foster mother because of her personal connection to the fos-ter care system:

[I have wanted to be a foster parent] I think as long as I can remember ... yeah. Because I know that a lot of these foster parents that kids get placed with should not be foster parents. ... Yeah, from my own experience, so I feel like at least I know that there will be one out there that I know for sure that, you know, is getting the kids because she loves kids and not just because she wants the check or, you know. ... And I know, you know, there is a couple other foster homes that we was in that was just really terrible ... and that I know should not have been foster parents. So I feel like, you know, like I said, I know that when I become a foster mother, this is what I want to do because I love kids and because I want to help them and because I don't want them being mis-treated. ... I remember telling myself that, you know, "When I grow up, I'm going to be a foster parent and, you know, make sure that these kids—kids will not be treated the way we were being treated." It was horrible. They took us away from our mother to put us in an even worse situation, you know.

Despite some of the women's desires to be foster mothers, none of the participants pursued this option during the study period, perhaps due to the complex bureaucracy of the foster care system or because the women of low SES were still waiting for a definitive "answer" regarding their childbearing difficulties before moving forward with a such a resolution (Hasenfeld 2010).

In addition to having more intimate knowledge of foster care than adoption, several other differences between the social mothering systems may have predisposed the participants toward one option over another. Adoption is costly, yet foster parents are paid for their services. The permanency of the relationship is also significantly different because many times foster children return to their biological parents. Additionally, although both prospective foster and adoptive parents are evaluated, the evaluation of prospective adoptive parents is more rigid and adheres more to mainstream ideas of what makes a good mother. Adoption also entails more paperwork and bureaucratic hurdles than does fostering, although prospective foster parents are still required to complete lengthy forms and course work.

For most women in the study, biological mothering is the preferred option, given stereotypical understandings of motherhood and family in the United States. When that option is not available, however, participants turn to forms of social mothering, such as adoption and foster care. Women of high SES are hesitant to choose those options, given their circumstances in which control is valued and foster care is unfamiliar. In contrast, women of low SES are open to such choices, but they face the same structural and financial barriers to adoption that are present in medical treatment for infertility.

Cultural beliefs about medicine and a history of negative encounters with physicians make women of low SES, particularly black women, hesitant to seek medical treatment for their infertility. Despite such negativity, the women of low SES still pursued medicine for an "answer" or diagnosis for their difficulties, but, as I have suggested, such a pursuit falls short, given medicine's inaccessibility to marginalized women. Medical institutions serve as a gatekeeper determining who should and who should not mother, or put another way, who should and who should not remain infertile. It is commonly recognized that economic inaccessibility excludes women of low SES from medical treatment for infertility. As sociologist Deborah Steinberg (1997, 45) observes, however, "to define reproductive choice/rights in terms of democratization of access to treatment would seem to assume that women's reproductive agency is both without and transcendent of context." The restrictive circumstances of economically disadvantaged women's lives, coupled with the classism that is an integral part of medicine, construct and constrain women's choices around reproductive health. The preferred way of achieving biological motherhood, medical treatment, is financially out of reach and inherently exclusionary. Yet the primary way to acquire social motherhood, adoption, is also a classed system.

In contrast to the exclusion of women of low SES, women of high SES are immersed in the medical experience. They plan the timeline of their treatments, select which doctor they will see, and then work with the physician to develop a treatment plan that suits their lifestyle and desires. Their demographic characteristics define them as good mothers, which relegates adoption to a "back pocket" option or last resort. Contrasting the classed experiences of resolving infertility ultimately exposes the intersection of the two institutions that control reproduction—motherhood and medicine—and how they maintain social norms regarding who can and cannot mother. The seemingly unlimited options to resolve childlessness among women of high SES compared to the limited choices of women of low SES determine how infertility affects their daily lives.

6

"So What Can You Do?"

• • • • • • • • • • • • • • • • • • • •

Coping with Infertility

> I'm at the point now where it's like,
> "Okay, I'm okay with if it doesn't hap-
> pen, I will be okay" because I don't really
> expect it to happen. Which in me, I have
> always—I have learned like a long time
> ago. I don't really expect a lot of things.
> —Carla, black woman of low SES

> I am pretty type A so [medicine] was
> something I could do. I could control
> that, I could go, I could do this, I could,
> you know, it was something I felt like
> that I was doing to get closer to my goal
> of getting pregnant.
> —Stacy, white woman of high SES

The infertility journey does not end with the choice (or lack thereof) of a resolution. The resolution itself greatly shapes how a woman experiences infertility. In particular, the participants' socioeconomic circumstances as well as whether or not they used medicine to resolve their infertility influenced how they coped with infertility and envisioned the future.

This final chapter of the infertility experience, however, is not captured in our current understanding of the condition. Most prior literature focuses on a cross section of the experience, typically when women are in the midst of it, such as when they are receiving medical care. Thus, post-infertility experiences, such as the effects of that care on the experience, go unexamined. Sociologist Peter Conrad concludes (1990, 1260), however, that to understand the complete illness experience we "must consider people's everyday lives lived *with* and *in spite of* illness."

Most medicalization literature is unable to thoroughly capture these components, given its lack of focus on race and class. As reproduction scholars note, "no research . . . has been done on whether women from different class locations make different choices about [reproductive] medical interventions, or perceive the procedures themselves or the information about procedures differently" (Dillaway and Brubaker 2006, 19). But previous chapters have revealed and other researchers have found that medicalization is indeed based in race and class ideas, which makes it all the more pertinent to examine how such demographic characteristics may or may not alter the process and effects of medicalization (Litt 1997; Steinberg 1997).

This chapter examines the final stages of an individual's journey through infertility. In doing so, I reveal how medicalization is refracted differently through the class structure and thus how class-based encounters with medicalization shape experiences of infertility. For instance, women of low SES, such as Carla, focus on coping with the experience of infertility, while women of high SES, such as Stacy, focus on coping with the medicalization of their infertility.

"I Don't Know Where to Go from Here": The Effects of Medical Exclusion and Inclusion

For most study participants, regardless of class, infertility is a devastating experience, but how that devastation plays out depends on context, including the presence of (other) stressors in one's life and the choice of resolution. The findings thus far demonstrate that social location does indeed differentially shape infertility experiences. The following results further that notion by exploring how the process of medicalization, as part of that social location, influences experience. Philosopher Michel Foucault (1975) demonstrated how the "clinical gaze" transforms an experience. Once an event is medicalized, much of its context is situated in medical institutions and worldviews, thereby impacting the way an individual interprets and reacts to the affliction. For the women in the study who received medical treatment for their infertility, namely those of high SES, medicine consumed their lives and shaped their coping mechanisms. In contrast, the remaining participants, primarily women of low SES who did not receive medical care for their infertility, faced limited options and were thus forced to put infertility on the "back burner."

As chapter 5 described, most women of low SES have limited, if any, access to medical resolutions for infertility. Their options are finite. Roberta, a white woman of low SES, laments, "I'll just keep doing what I'm doing. And I think there's nothing else I can do." Jewel, a white woman of low SES, echoes Roberta's stalemate:

> I just—I know there's something wrong and I just—there's nothing I can do to figure out what is wrong with me . . . And that's very hard to know that there's people out there that could tell me what's wrong with me but it's all about money. And that drives me crazy how this world is about money when you could help me and figure out so I could have a baby and you can't. That's just not happening. . . . Honestly I don't know where to go from here. I'm going to try to see about getting this doctor and everything, but other than that, there's no—no other place I can go to unless if I fall into a bunch of money and I can go have this done.

Such limitations force women of low SES to cope with their infertility rather than dwell on its presence or solutions. In effect, women of low SES try to dissociate themselves and their lives from their infertility. Barbara, a tall, black woman of low SES, explains: "But I don't allow myself really to think, think, think about it because I can't do anything about it, you know. I wish that things were different and, you know, it just doesn't happen." Barbara does not allow herself to think about her fertility difficulties because she cannot do anything about them.

Having to move on with life may be particularly necessary for women of low SES, given the other obligations and responsibilities that require their full attention. Judy, a white woman of low SES, describes: "I mean it's an isolated kind of thing because at that point you also have other responsibilities and most people we have jobs, you know, we have other responsibilities and responses and things like that." For women of low SES, infertility becomes an "isolated" event in their lives in which other responsibilities take precedence. Women of low SES can literally not afford to focus on something they are unable to resolve. Additionally, women of low SES may be more apt to move on with their lives because they are used to loss and lacking control over life events. One study found that while middle-class women experience infertility as a foreclosure of choice, women of low SES, who have endured other hardships in life, experience infertility more in terms of general adversity and less in terms of control (Heitman 1995).

While women of low SES face finite options to resolve their infertility, medicalization produces the opposite effect for women of high SES. The seemingly infinite treatment options available to women of high SES have their own repercussions. Infertility is a unique "illness" in that treatment ends only when the patient chooses for it to cease. Although there is a limited number of procedures available to treat infertility, those procedures can be repeated until either funds expire or a woman can no longer handle the emotional and physical intensity they require (Zoll 2013). It is difficult for women of high SES, in particular, to stop pursuing treatment because of their circumstances in which they are used to setting and meeting goals. Thus, quitting rather than persisting with treatment is more difficult for them to accomplish. In other words, in addition to the burden infertility places upon an individual, women receiving medical treatment have the "burden of not trying hard enough" if they do not exhaust all treatment options (Shattuck and Schwarz 1991, 335).

For women of high SES, the choice of medical treatment for infertility may not be a choice at all. Indeed, Colleen, a white woman of high SES, reflects such sentiments: "This is like a drug. It is very much like a drug. You get a little bit and you don't get what you need out of it and you need more. And it's addicting. I mean you—you get so close and you find out there's this one more thing that might get you what you want. And you—you're like, 'Well, I've got to try this one more thing. I have tried so much, why not try one more thing?' So I knew when we were doing IUIs that there was no way I could give up there."

Colleen perceives that she was "addicted" to medically treating her infertility. The "infertility treadmill" or "rollercoaster," as it is often termed, is specific to women of high SES who are constantly on the ups and downs of hormone treatments and receiving encouragement and letdown with each new procedure and each new failure that may ensue. Such experiences starkly contrast with that relayed by Jewel who was frustrated with her infertility because she could not do anything about it.

Nadia, a white woman of high SES, further describes the seemingly never-ending options available for medically treating infertility:

> It's usually in the beginning, you know, you're kind of—you're very upset but you're also hopeful. You're frustrated and bitter but you still have that hope and you're like, "Hey, it's just matter of time. You know, I've just got to control." And then you wait and wait and it doesn't happen. "Well, next cycle. You know, they say that this is just the first, you know, because there's—we're on plan B. You know, there's like A to Z. And this didn't work, no problem. We'll go to C and we'll go to D." So you keep going through that and, you know, you try to not get discouraged but each mo—each month it becomes harder. You know, it doesn't become really easier for a while. . . . And you go through all of these things and it's exhausting. Totally exhausting. And you get to the point where you can't humanly do any more. And it's still not happening. So that's when it gets really kind of—that's when you kind of hit bottom. And, you know, I—I kind of—and I have even taken a break and stopped with the Western medicine and gone to Eastern medicine for three months. I just saw an acupuncturist and took herbs and that didn't work. I didn't even get a period with all of the strong herbs and acupuncture and everything. So I went back to Western medicine and, you know, it's hard because, you know, it's like during those now it's three years.

Nadia provides a detailed picture of the infinite options available to women of high SES. Not only did she access "A to Z" medical treatment options, but when she was unsatisfied with their results she pursued Eastern medicine in Canada that, according to her, was "very costly." These pursuits have consumed three years of Nadia's life, and she is still not done:

> So I'm not looking forward to [IVF] and I'm just really terrified. Because that's it. And then after that, I don't know. I mean I guess there's still options. After that, if IVF doesn't work, we'll probably try it again but I wouldn't try it in the same clinic unless I had leftover eggs because I don't know if the clinic that I'm going to is the best. There is a like wonder clinic in Colorado that a lot of

people go to. Actually I know somebody who had two failed IVFs here and went to Colorado and got pregnant. So I'd probably go there. If that didn't work, then I'd go to India . . . and they actually have different things that they have tried and actually some of the medicine's even ironically more advanced there.

As Nadia's story demonstrates, the possibilities for medically treating infertility are endless (for women of high SES).

While women of low SES attempted to push their infertility experiences from the center of their lives, women of high SES had infertility consume their lives through the effects of medical care. Barbara could not afford to "think, think, think" about her infertility, but women of high SES, inundated in medical treatment, are forced to constantly think about their infertility. Carole, a white woman of high SES, explains: "[I think about infertility] a lot. A lot. And then even when you know it's not time, you're thinking about the next time and what you're going to do to make it better and right. Surely this will be the time. And you're just going through the days. That's very true, too. You're just going through the days to get to the next time and when you have another chance. And, you know, that seems kind of sad, too. You know, I felt like I was just going through the motions of life for a while." Carole and other women of high SES thought about their infertility so much that they "just went through the motions of life for a while."

In addition to mental exhaustion, medically treating infertility physically consumed actual time in high SES women's days, commitments that resulted in drastic life changes. For example, Colleen, a white woman of high SES, quit her job to accommodate the rigorous schedule required of her medical treatments:

But the—the other interesting thing or the other thing that, you know, just really happened at this point was just the absolute control it has over your life. Because, you know, on day one, you call and then on day three you have to go in and, you know, even though I pretty much knew my cycle, day one give or take a day, well, that makes a difference. Especially if you're looking at a weekend and so people would ask us to go places and we would say, "You know, I don't know if I can because I might have to go to the hospital that day for blood work" or—I mean and that was—that was constant. At that point on from the time we went to Fertility University on, that was a constant thing.

You know, because you just don't really ever know. And people don't understand that at all.

Similarly, Stacy, a white woman of high SES, altered her work schedule in order to continue her infertility treatments: "I said, 'I have to be able to focus on this and we're going to a doctor and we, you know, this is really important to me.' And when I need to have a, you know, just a slower schedule right now so I can get into these appointments and not worry about like how I'm going to find that four or five hours. . . . And so I went down to three days a week during that time so I could kind of do my—my—the doctor I needed to do and it wasn't always the same days of the week because when they needed to see you depended on, you know, the whole cycle of the month." Stacy went from working as a full-time lawyer to working part-time in order to accommodate the frequent, rigid medical appointments required of infertility treatment. Women of high SES were in positions in which they could make such life-altering changes, unlike women of low SES.

Infertile women are often stereotyped as "desperate." Unlike the media's portrayal, however, in which desperateness is portrayed as the reason for pursuing medical treatment for infertility, the findings indicate that the treatment itself causes the despair to ensue. As Sarah Franklin (1992) reflects, "It is the hope IVF gives which can cause the desperation it is said to alleviate." In other words, the "desperate" infertile label primarily applies to treatment-seekers, most of whom are women of high SES.

Whether or not a woman receives medical treatment for infertility shapes her experience. Women of low SES are forced to move on with their lives, whereas high SES women's lives are consumed by thoughts and procedures surrounding infertility.

Coping with Infertility

But *how* do the women of low SES move on with their lives, and *how* do the women of high SES cope with the inundation of medicine? These groups have different coping mechanisms and strategies, yet all women are active, agentic players in the process. This finding is counter to much of the current understanding about coping responses between social classes. Literature typically portrays women of low SES as passive and fatalistic and women of high SES as more active and controlling in their responses to life events (Zadoroznyj 1999). Portraying the socioeconomic groups in such a manner, however, results in a binary, dichotomous way of thinking about life reactions, but these are not mutually exclusive categories. Indeed, being fatalistic does not prevent agency (Bell 2009; Bell 2010).

Some women use fatalistic statements as a way to cope with health outcomes; in other words, fatalism becomes agentic (Bolam et al. 2003; Keeley, Wright, and Condit 2009). This is particularly true for women of low SES who live in circumstances with few resources that allow them to control life events. For example, Ruby, a white woman of low SES, reflects on the lack of options she faces to resolve her infertility and offers fatalistic statements, yet she also demonstrates how she is able to "get through it," which requires a more active role: "[I] keep on trucking one day at a time. I don't—I'm not—it's not going to bother me unless something major goes on and it comes up or we have a conver—my husband and I have another conversation and then I lose my cool every time. . . . So we'll get through it I think. . . . It's either [grow] or, you know, keep going in a bad path and nothing's ever going to change. And I'd rather change for better instead of worse. So what can you do? You can't do nothing."

Even though Ruby believes that she "can't do" anything about her infertility, she and the other women of low SES in the study have numerous coping strategies and mechanisms that they utilize in order to "grow" and make "change." Some of the women of low SES are not yet ready to stop pursuing pregnancy and seek ways to resolve their childlessness. They primarily do this in two ways (Bell 2010). First, some women, unaware of structural constraints, primarily concentrate on overcoming the economic barriers to medical treatment. Second, other participants, aware of their exclusion from infertility treatments, avoid medicine altogether and derive alternative, nonmedical techniques to resolve their childlessness.

Some participants attempt to surmount the financial constraints of infertility treatment by deriving innovative ways to pay for the services. Doing so may overcome their (economic) exclusion from medicine; however, the structural barriers remain. Unlike the unique ways individuals of high SES have reported to accumulate money (Greil 1991), such as remortgaging their homes, these opportunities may not be available to individuals of lower economic standing who do not own such assets. Instead, women of low SES must develop creative ways to utilize the limited resources at hand. Sherry, a white woman of low SES in her early thirties, reflects: "[My husband's] got like if you see out there a bunch of old Camaros and, you know, and he had like somebody came out and like assessed his cars and stuff and he's got like $1.2 million in cars. He—yeah, old cars. He's got old cars everywhere. But, you know, it came to a point to where, you know, this is—this is what we decided to do. For the next year we're going to try and if it doesn't happen, he's going to take one of his old cars and he's going to sell it and we're going to go do in vitro (laughs)." Sherry suggests selling one or more of her husband's cars as a way to pay for IVF. They are willing to part with a hobby as well as their property to seek medical treatment for infertility.

Carrie, a white woman of low SES, and her partner similarly make sacrifices to try to finance fertility treatment. Carrie left home at age sixteen and did not communicate with her mother for the next decade. However, after reconciling, Carrie decided to let her mother who had recently lost her home live with her and her partner in their trailer home: "[My partner is] a bus driver (laughing). We are poor. . . . My mom just went through a divorce after twenty-one years and it wasn't mutual and it was devastating and so he got the house and she wasn't ready to buy a house. And so she moved in with us. And she was going to give us $1,000 a month. So then I was hoping she would stay for a year and so then that's IVF."

While giving her mother a place to stay seems commendable, Carrie describes this choice as solely made on the basis of earning money for IVF. In fact, Carrie told me that she is charging her mother much more than she would any other tenant as a ploy to make money faster. Carrie's plan was unsuccessful; she became unemployed and had to use the money from her mother for living expenses rather than savings for infertility treatment. Changed circumstances forced Carrie to revise her solution:

ANN: So how long do you think it will be until you can afford IVF?

CARRIE: I think that I want to save half of it and then just go in debt for the other half. Because that seems more manageable than (pauses)—I don't— we're just so—we—we just—we live debt free, you know. So us going into debt is like a big deal. And we don't have the option of taking out a second mortgage on our house or, you know, other people do. I don't even know if I could get a loan. I am just assuming that I can. I have no idea.

Without options that "other people" have, Carrie is forced to go into debt, a position she has not been in before. She has run out of other solutions to her infertility, and "there's nowhere to go but IVF."

Despite all the creativity and time spent thinking about ways to afford medical treatment, particularly IVF, only one participant of low SES, Laura, actually received IVF services. The procedure, a "gift" from her boyfriend who eventually became her husband, was unsuccessful, and she eventually adopted two children. The lack of medical care among the participants reflects the difficulty of attaining monetary resources to afford infertility treatments coupled with potential structural and political barriers the women of low SES confront in their medical pursuits.

The participants, however, did not only pursue medical resolutions to their childlessness. Perhaps conscious of their exclusion from infertility treatment, the women of low SES develop alternative, nonmedical solutions to resolving their childlessness (Bell 2009). Donna, a black woman of low SES, attempts to rub pregnant women's stomachs in hopes of achieving conception: "Yeah, but it's supposed to be good luck if you rub (both laugh) . . . I do that a lot (both laughing). I do that a whole lot, yeah. I can see a pregnant woman on the street and I'll be like, 'Please, can I rub your stomach? It's supposed to be good luck.'" Employing folk methods was commonplace among the participants. Carrie, a white woman of low SES, tried "everything she [heard]" from "doing a few things like raspberry leaf tea . . . to eating an Egg McMuffin."

In addition to trying to achieve biological motherhood through medical and nonmedical means, the women crafted ways to achieve social motherhood to resolve their childlessness. This echoes one researcher's (Parry 2005b) finding that infertile women extend their understandings of family beyond the traditional ideology focused on biological children. For economically disadvantaged women, however, options for such extension are limited, owing to the classist basis of adoption. Given this exclusion, women turn to other forms of social mothering. Several of the women of low SES in this study undertook the primary role of stepmother to fulfill their mothering desires. Heather, a biracial woman of low SES, reconciles her infertility in this manner:

ANN: So if you were to outline the next five or ten years of your life, which of those options, [adoption, IVF, or stepmothering], do you think will pan out?

HEATHER: I think it's the step-mom because my husband and I have talked about him taking full custody, you know, of his younger son just due to the situation he's in. And I think that comes from wanting to be a mom plus not

liking the situation he's in and if we could give him better, why are we not?
I think we're obligated, you know, to give him better so he can do better.

In deciding how to resolve her infertility, Heather chooses stepmothering over adoption or IVF. Perhaps knowing she cannot access the latter options, Heather prioritizes the one that is most attainable. She justifies this decision based on the notion that she "can do it better" than the children's biological mother.

Taking care of others is a dominant theme around motherhood; hence, many participants negotiate the infertility experience through this action (Hays 1996). Jackie, a white woman of low SES, explains:

> I'm just trying to fill something and like with my brother coming to live with us, I think maybe we asked him because I wanted somebody else to take care of. You know, my mom said that once he starts college, he can't stay with us but at the same time, I feel like if he leaves, then it's just back to me taking care of my husband, you know. And I—it's not that I don't love that. I want to take care of my husband but I just—he's not there all the time and so, you know, he works a lot of hours. And so I just—I'm trying to fill it with other things and I shouldn't be.

Jackie is able to mother in the sense that she is taking care of someone other than her husband. Not only does this allow her to attain a salient characteristic of motherhood, but it also relieves her loneliness in her husband's absence.

Candace, a black woman of low SES, also extends the ideology of motherhood to include experiences beyond biological children. After struggling with infertility for years, Candace had a hysterectomy following cervical cancer, a surgery that eliminated any prior hopes she had for having her own children. The following reflects how she coped with and negotiated this realization:

> ANN: So how did you feel after all of that: knowing that now you probably wouldn't have kids without a miracle?
>
> CANDACE: Just like—it's just like God to me because a lot of people are coming to me with, "You can do everything. You—you can still be a mother. You can take care of other children [by teaching] young girls to not go down the

path I went down in the negative sense to drugs and alcohol." So I could be like a mother. . . . So that's what (crying) I'm going to do.

Candace can "be like a mother" in ways that extend beyond biological children, yet encompass normalized characteristics of motherhood, such as caretaking.

Although stepmothering and caretaking are not limited to women of low SES, they are more prevalent among such groups. According to the National Survey of Family Growth, nearly 21 percent of women with less than a high school education have cared for a nonbiological child, including stepchildren and children of other kin, compared with 8 percent of women with at least a college degree (Chandra et al. 2005). Thus, the women of low SES in this study, with limited resolutions to childlessness, adopt roles typically associated with their economic status; they in turn, maintain the hierarchy, or stratification, that exists around motherhood (Glenn 2010).

With limited options, many women of low SES turn to religion to cope with their childlessness. Contrary to popular thinking, however, religion is not merely used as a defensive, passive response to life events. Such a view is overly simplistic and based on stereotypes (Geertz 1973; Pargament and Park 1995). Instead, religion can be active as well as passive, assertive as well as defensive; religion allows women to actively reconstruct and reinterpret negative events more positively (Ellison et al. 2001). Angie, a black woman of low SES, demonstrates such agentic use of religion: "Ah, God has gave me a lot of strength. Going to church and just praying about it (pauses) has gave me strength. Just—just keeping hope in general and just keeping hope and just hoping, you know, I can have kids and this has got me through." Angie purposefully sought out religion to cope with her infertility by attending church and praying; this practice brought her hope and thus allowed her to "get through" the perils of infertility.

The participants are situated in a dilemma; deriving ways to pay for medical treatment does not overcome the structural barriers the women face in medicine (for example, the appointment structure), yet developing alternative solutions furthers their exclusion from the institution of motherhood. In turn, women of low SES, as Heather describes, are forced to "come to grips" and cope with their inability to conceive and move on with their life goals. Many women of low SES cope with their infertility by changing their attitudes toward it. They shift from thinking "it is not the right time" to thinking "it is not meant to be," a change that allows them to move on with their lives. Although both thoughts have fatalistic undertones, the women use such mentality as a coping mechanism.

Communications scholar Bethany Keeley and her colleagues (2009) found that fatalistic talk many times results from women realizing that certain life events are beyond their control. When faced with such constraints, talking positively gives them a sense of control or agency. In the case of infertility, women of low SES have far less control due to the limited resources available to them in their environments compared to women of high SES, which results in more fatalistic statements among them. It is one of their only ways to cope. Tanya, a white woman of low SES, reflects: "I didn't—I would just say, 'It's just not the right time.' And I didn't want to say, 'It was not meant to be' yet because I wasn't really quite done yet. So that says—when I was thirty-four or thirty-five, I just said, 'You know, it's just—it's not meant to be.' So I kind of resolved myself that, 'All right, forget about it and just move on.'"

Carla, a black woman of low SES, similarly "moves on" with her life by changing the way she thinks about her infertility: "Like now I go through without even like, 'If it happens, it happens. If it don't, it don't.' No. I'm at the point now where it's like, 'Okay, I'm okay with if it doesn't happen, I will be okay' because I don't really expect it to happen. Which in me, I have always—I have learned like a long time ago. I don't really expect a lot of things. So—because if you expect them and it doesn't happen, you feel worse. So if you just don't expect them to happen and just like (gasps), 'Oh, okay!'"

Jessica, a white woman of low SES in her late thirties, also alters her mindset: "Okay, everything that I have gone through is hard and bad but, you know, I mean somewhere somehow, there's somebody that has worse. You know, it's like I still have a great—I mean I have so much. I am blessed with what I have got. It's like, 'Be happy for what you have and not so much what you can't have.' You know, things don't always work exactly the way we dream and plan. So but they work. So and—and like I said, I believe everything happens for a reason so somehow, some way it's going to be better."

The coping strategies of both Carla and Jessica demonstrate how it might be easier for women of low SES to deal with their infertility compared to women of high SES. As Carla says, they have learned "not to expect a lot of things" in their lives, and, as Jessica adds, many women of low SES know others in much more dire straits than their experiences of childlessness. Given their restrictive surroundings, low SES women's perspectives about infertility shift and allow them to cope with their childlessness.

While women of low SES concentrate their efforts on coping with infertility itself, women of high SES focus on coping with the medicalization of their infertility. As Colleen relayed, medical treatment for infertility "controls" your life, so women of high SES, who live in a context in which control is paramount, focus on regaining that control. One way in which the women of high SES attempt to do so is through in-depth research of infertility, as Nadia explains:

> I feel so out of control and I wish someone would just swoop in and say, "Nadia, everything's going to be all right." And [my husband] says it but not like—I just almost wish someone would take control and take the burden off of me in some way. So yeah. [I regain control] by reading too much about fertility. But that only took me so far and then it just kind of after a while it's like a diminishing returns and then it just makes it worse. So then I have read all I can and I know all I need to know and any more is just going to depress me. And so I think I try to, you know, be a control freak in other ways of life and that helps me. But then I found that that just stresses me out so . . . it's a whole emotional cycle. Like a development. It kind of happens when you're going through this and it kind of leads you ironically to like let go of a lot of control because you're so helpless.

After three years of trying to "control" her infertility in various ways, infertility taught Nadia that she cannot control everything in life. Indeed, Nadia "let go of a lot of control," which helped her cope with feelings of helplessness.

Many women of high SES turn to medicine to try to control their infertility. In doing so, they lose more control over their reproduction and their lives (Greil et al. 2011a). Unconscious of such effects, however, women of high SES, such as Stacy, seek medicine to stabilize their lives:

> I am pretty type A so [medicine] was something I could do. I could control that, I could go, I could do this, I could, you know, it was something I felt like

that I was doing to get closer to my goal of getting pregnant. . . . So in that sense I do think it helped. . . . You know, and but it was also reassuring like, "I am here with this doctor and they can do all of these great things and look at all of these people they're getting pregnant and look at how they're going to increase our chance of success. And if we were just, you know, on our own trying, our chances would be this. But now with this drug and with this treatment and with this procedure, like we're just increasing our chances." So in that sense I think it helped because I felt like I was taking steps and that it was—and so I was taking more control over like making it happen and (pauses) . . .

The hope that medicine provides causes women to seek its assistance. Taking the action to do so allowed Stacy to feel like she was more in control over her infertility because it was her choice. She also felt reassured by her decision to seek medicine because of its "high success rate." Ironically, it is precisely this hope in medicine that causes more desperation and angst among the women's experiences because it pressures them to continue seeking medical assistance. In reality, the "high success rate" to which Stacy refers may be falsely perceived (Zoll 2013). According to the most recent report from the Centers for Disease Control and Prevention (CDC), less than 30 percent of ART cycles resulted in a live birth in 2010 (Centers for Disease Control and Prevention 2013b). In other words, there is a high likelihood that infertility treatment will *not* work, thereby causing the cycle of more treatment and loss of control to continue.

Some women of high SES turned to their occupations to cope with their feelings of helplessness. Nan describes her coping strategy: "And so I started my own business. . . . That gave me a sense of purpose and a feeling of being in—in control of something in my life and—and, you know, built up a clientele and, you know, taught cooking classes and got a lot of fulfillment from that. It felt—it felt like I was doing something that I enjoyed, that was helping other people and I was getting good feedback from others, you know, that—who appreciated what I was doing. . . . So that helped me to feel a little more control of my life." For Nan, starting her own business was not only a way to regain control of her life, but it also provided her with a "sense of purpose." Pronatalism and the motherhood mandate construct motherhood as women's purpose in life. Thus, when motherhood is not achieved, women must find other sources of meaning. Work gave the women a sense of self-worth outside motherhood, which allowed them to cope with their infertility.

Some women turned to solutions to stabilize their lives, but they had detrimental effects on their health. In addition to starting a new job, Nan looked to food to help her feelings of powerlessness: "I had a hard—hard time just dealing with life on life's terms and so, you know, the infertility was part of one of those things that I just had a hard time dealing with. And for me I guess I tried to, you know, I couldn't control this and so I, 'Well, at least I can eat,' you know, even though it was self-sabotaging." Nan's compulsive eating disorder, a mechanism to cope with her infertility, allowed her to feel in control of something in her life, despite its negative health effects. After eight years since starting her infertility journey, Nan is still recuperating from her eating disorder.

Different ways of resolving infertility led to differences in how the women coped with their childlessness. Women of low SES concentrate on overcoming their childlessness and ultimately coming to terms with its "reality." Women of high SES, however, do not focus so much on infertility itself; rather, they focus on coping with their lack of control over the experience.

"Look at All of the Options": Future Goals

Such socioeconomic differences in coping cause the women to have different visions of their futures. Despite the limited options to resolve their infertility, some women of low SES still envision having children at some point in their lives. For instance, Jewel, a white woman of low SES, describes what will happen in the next five years of her life: "I'm going to get married. I am going to have everything set. I want all of my bills paid and I want to be able to take care of everything. I don't want to have a lot of stress in my life. I am going to live it to the fullest and I'm going to try to have one more baby. Whether I can have one, two, three, as long as they'll stay alive. I don't care how many I'll have. But after that if it doesn't work, then I'm not going to ever try again . . . I'm just going to put it on the back burner." After having several miscarriages, Jewel is going to try to have one more baby, but first she wants to stabilize her life through marriage, debt reduction, and stress management. As discussed in chapter 2, women of low SES believe that having a stable life (regardless of income) is important in determining an individual's readiness to be a good mother. Jewel believes that by achieving such readiness she establishes a higher likelihood of having a successful pregnancy.

Similarly, Ebony, a black woman of low SES, hopes for increased stability in the near future so that she can continue trying to have children: "Well, [in the next five years] I see myself becoming a professional certified pharmacist. And I feel like when I get back into a new professional career, I can pursue the kids. But right now I just feel like everything is just going to just get better and better and better. If kids come in play with that, then I'll have kids. But right now, everything is pretty good." Like Jewel, Ebony wants to have a stable job before trying to have children again. Focusing on one's self in such a manner was a much more prominent theme in low SES women's visions of the future than those among women of high SES. Lacking options and being forced to deal with their infertility may allow the women of low SES to more easily focus on individual, personal goals that go beyond mothering (which contrasts with their peers, as elucidated in chapter 4).

Heather, a biracial woman of low SES, exemplifies this idea: "But it's more of, 'Look at all of the options you've got. Look at all of the things that you're doing or that you can do that you enjoy.' So I think as my life has changed and I have looked at all of these other things I am able to do now and we have talked about moving out of state and stuff like that. And so it's like, 'Why not? Why just limit yourself to wanting to be a mom and having kids when life has so many more things to offer than just that?'" Roberta, a white woman of low SES, echoes Heather's sentiments when she describes what will happen in the next five years: "Finishing my master's. Getting a job teaching. Settling in somewhere and maybe even buying a house because we haven't done that yet. But that would be about it. Just, you know, going on with life." Roberta, an aspiring actress, will "go on with life" by focusing on herself rather than concentrating on her childlessness.

When asked to outline the next five years of their lives, some women of low SES had a difficult time doing so. Their economic circumstances, which cause life to be unpredictable and in which control is less achievable, make discussing the future impossible for some participants. Ruby, a white woman of low SES, explains:

ANN: Well, if you were to outline the next five years of your life, how do you see it playing out?

RUBY: I don't know. I can't give you an answer to that one anymore. Because five years ago, we put up our Christmas tree this year and every year we have—we buy new Christmas ornaments and one year we were so broke that I made stockings out of scrapbooking paper and on the back I asked my husband to put down five things that he wanted in the next five years. And I did one and he did one and we looked at 'em this year and our five years are up and we wanted a house, you know, or—I'm thinking of his. He wants a house, he wants some kind of car, he wants children, he wants a garage, and something else. And out of all of these things on our lists, none of them came true. So I really can't even tell you that anymore because after seeing that and acknowledging that, "Wow, we didn't accomplish anything in five years," felt really horrible. "So we're just about five years off I think, Clyve. I don't know what else to tell you, Buddy. Sorry." So.

Used to not getting things in life, women of low SES are hesitant to predict a future that might not "come true."

Women of high SES outline similar futures in that they also hope to have children, and they, too, have a difficult time envisioning what the future entails. Their class circumstances, however, shape and alter the reasoning behind such predictions. As Nan states, "We never considered just being—accepting childlessness. That was just not something either one of us wanted." Although both socioeconomic groups wanted more children in their futures, women of high SES were much more determined to make such a goal happen compared to women of low SES who, like Ebony, were "good" if it did not happen and would just "put it on the backburner," as Jewel described. High SES women's determination was typically pursued through continual use of medical treatment so many of the higher-class women's visions of the future were mainly filled with doctors' offices. Brooke demonstrates:

Well, at some point in the next five years, I will have had at least one child. I really—I really think we'll have more than one by then 'cuz I still I have this feeling somewhere deep inside that part of me tries to suppress because I don't want to let posit—I am afraid to let positive thoughts surface too much because if I think too positively, then I just get crushed more. It's more of a let down. I am not as negative as I was when I was in that dark period but I'm—I'm afraid to be a super, bubbly, upbeat, positive person. But I do have this just deep-seated thought that somewhere, somehow we will figure out how to get pregnant. I am not sure if we'll have to go through invasive treatments or not. But whatever that way is, we'll figure it out and we'll be able to use that same avenue to have future children.

Brooke was certain that in the next five years she "will have had at least one child." Such confidence greatly contrasts with the hesitancy inherent in the low SES women's future predictions, in which having a child "might" or "possibly could" happen. The differences in tone and semantics reflect class variations in control over life events, and they also demonstrate why moving on with life may be an easier task for women of low SES compared to their high SES counterparts. Knowing that it might not happen allows the women to accept that possibility and focus on other aspects of their lives.

Part of the certitude voiced by women of high SES stems from the confidence placed in medicine. Science and technology are portrayed as infallible, and medicine is believed to provide a "cure" for all things health-related. Thus, medical treatments for infertility give women hope and assurance that their childlessness will be resolved (Zoll 2013). Colleen, a white woman of high SES, reflects on the hope it provides:

I—I mean I—I hope—I—I do think we'll have another [child]. I do think that we'll try for this, you know, use these frozen embryos and try for one more. Which is a very difficult decision given my age. That's what worries me the most. Just thinking about it eighteen years from now. But—but I do think we will do that. And interestingly enough, in my mind, I'm thinking, "We will most certainly get pregnant." I mean like when I think about, "Are we going to do it or not?" it's, "Are we going to have another baby?" It's not, "Are we going to try this again?" I definitely in my mind I'm thinking, "Of course this is going to work. This is a great batch of embryos."

Colleen and other women of high SES are confident that children will be in their futures due to both social norms centering on control as well as their access to medical treatments for infertility, both of which are absent from the lives of women of low SES.

Similar to Ruby, women of high SES also have a difficult time predicting their futures; however, unlike Ruby who was unable to outline her future due to her working-class lifestyle in which predictability and control over life events is infrequent, women of high SES can no longer envision their futures because of the lack of control that infertility has introduced into their lives. For example, infertility is the first time in Nadia's life that things have not gone according to plan:

> I don't know. That's the big void that I don't know. That's why—see, I've only seen myself [as a mother] my whole life. So not seeing myself that way, it's like that's why—that kind of is it hits now in the head in where I am right now with for the first time in my life I don't have a place where I'm going. I'm not going to where I see my life heading. I don't know where it's going. I'm just kind of there. Whatever comes, then I guess I'm just leaving it up to God or fate or whatever because I don't know. The only thing I can even picture is almost so extreme that it's almost fanciful rather than realistic. It's like just chucking everything and just going and being a nomad and maybe doing some spiritual things in India or joining the Peace Corps or something, you know?

Nadia is unable to control her fertility, a realization that leaves her help-less and lost in "fanciful" notions. Rather than focusing on life's next steps, like Heather's plans for vacations and school, women of high SES, as Sarah states, "no longer think that way anymore." Women of high SES are lit-erally unable to plan for their futures because they have lost their previ-ous ability to control life events. Planning and controlling were more than mere characteristics; they were embedded within the identities of women of high SES. Thus, infertility caused women of high SES to lose not only the motherhood aspect of their identities but also the controlling, predict-able aspect of their lives.

The experience of infertility is truly a never-ending journey, yet how women learn to cope and live with infertility is largely determined by their economic circumstances and the way in which they resolve it, either medi-cally or not. The options available to resolve infertility coupled with the prevalence and ability to control life events greatly shape how women of different classes confront infertility and how they envision their futures.

The limited options available to women of low SES to resolve their infer-tility force them to "not think" about it and move on with life. As Roberta questions, "What else [are they] supposed to do?" However, for women receiving medical treatments for their infertility, primarily women of high SES, infertility consumes their lives, largely due to the nature of the treat-ments. The hope medicine provides and its rigorous treatment schedule combined with the cultural practice of "not quitting" in high SES settings cause women to perpetually pursue treatment and its "A-to-Z" options.

Such differences in options and solutions to infertility cause variations in how women of different classes cope with infertility. Women of low SES focus more on getting over the experience of infertility itself while women of high SES concentrate on regaining control of their lives and coping with the inundation of medicine. Both groups' coping mechanisms are agentic, active, and purposeful, but, for women of low SES, many times their circumstances limit their coping abilities to more fatalistic responses, such as prayer and attitude.

Ultimately, the experience of infertility has shaped how women envision their futures. Women of low SES, used to not having things go their way, are able to envision a life beyond infertility and strive to attain personal goals, such as further education or more travel. Women of high SES, however, are unable to make such a transition. They can either no longer predict their futures, or they can only envision more medical treatments to achieve their goal of biological motherhood. In other words, women of low SES are able to live *with* infertility while women of high SES are determined to *overcome* it, and, until they do, they cannot envision a life at all.

Conclusion

· ·

(Re)conceiving Infertility

"I don't think infertility is a problem. Usually it's the other way around—[women of low SES are having too many children]," a woman from a social service agency told me as I inquired about recruiting participants from her facility. Although I was aware that stereotypes of infertility existed, I quickly learned just how ingrained such ideas are—even agencies serving women of low SES did not recognize the presence of infertility among their clients. Throughout the book we learn how such stereotypes shape experiences of infertility and, even more important, how those mainstream ideas are rooted in ideological notions of motherhood, family, and health. Notions of who should mother, how families should be arranged, and who should access medical treatments both shape and are shaped by our understandings of fertility and reproduction. In short, class matters in shaping infertility; examining why and how class matters begins to reveal the social basis of infertility.

Why and How Class Matters

The entire journey of the infertility experience varies among women of different social classes—from before they realize they are infertile and just beginning to think about motherhood to the strategies they use to resolve infertility. What are some of the reasons for this difference? In other words, *why* does social class matter when thinking about infertility?

Quite simply, women of different classes live in different contexts, and the social practices and messages in those contexts vary across class groups. For instance, women of low SES approach pregnancy more fatalistically and "naturally" compared to the high SES women's planned, organized, and mechanical ways of "trying" to become pregnant. These differences shape how and when the women come to realize they have childbearing difficulties. Women of low SES take longer to recognize their childbearing difficulties due to their less "planful" approaches to pregnancy. Additionally, women of low SES are more likely than women of high SES to have children at younger ages, less likely to marry, and more likely to avoid talking to others about personal problems. The lack of a committed partner coupled with fewer peers they can relate to cause women of low SES to have less support for their childbearing difficulties.

One of the more obvious reasons class matters is money. Unable to afford medical treatment for infertility, women of low SES are forced to seek alternative, nonmedical ways to resolve their childlessness, but women of low SES face barriers to medical treatment that go well beyond the financial. Discrimination, time constraints, and insurance limitations are just a few of the barriers women of low SES confront in the health care system—barriers most women of high SES do not encounter. Whether a woman resolves her infertility medically or nonmedically influences how she copes with her childlessness and projects her future. Women of low SES, not inundated in the seemingly infinite options of medicine, are able to focus on getting over the experience of infertility, while women of high SES are more concerned about coping with the lack of control they have over the medical treatment itself.

These differences in the infertility experience are rooted in the very different social locations of the women in this study. Important similarities in the infertility experience, however, should also be mentioned. First, infertility was devastating to all women it affected. It disrupted every aspect of their lives, from their identity as mothers to their future aspirations. Yet all participants, regardless of socioeconomic group, actively attempted to confront their childlessness. For instance, women of low SES devised alternative ways to try to become pregnant, while women of high SES actively researched the best physicians, practices, and treatments. Along with such activism, however, both groups also had fatalistic, or more passive, reactions to their reproductive struggles. This was especially apparent for women of low SES because they were constrained by the cultural and material resources available to them, but, as time elapsed, participants of high SES also resigned themselves to face protracted struggles with infertility. As Nadia told me, "[Infertility] kind of leads you ironically to like let go of a lot of control because you're so helpless. . . . I have totally changed the way I look at my life. I really don't care about anything anymore. I am just kind of trying to live in the moment."

In thinking about these findings, it is important to recognize the limits of the study. I focused on class diversity for several reasons, as outlined in my introduction. In doing so, I focused less on gender, age, sexuality, and race diversity. I chose to only examine women's experiences of infertility as opposed to couples' or men's experiences for several reasons. First, infertility is typically viewed as a woman's issue due to the gendered nature of reproduction and parenting. For this reason, researchers have found that infertility is more salient in the lives of women than men (Greil 1991). Second, most infertility research is conducted on women, but women of a certain type—white, wealthy women. Limiting this study to women, albeit a more diverse group of women, allowed me to both converse with *and* fill a significant gap in the current research on infertility. Finally, holding gender constant allows for a more nuanced examination of class differences in infertility. Despite these advantages, future research should examine the gender dynamics of infertility. Infertility provides an ideal case for exploring the relationship of gender to an individual's reproductive capacity. Men's infertility, in particular, needs further examination. By failing to study men's responses to infertility, researchers reinforce the construction of infertility as a woman's issue.

Focusing on class also limited my emphasis on racial diversity. Although race is not predominant in infertility research, when diversity is examined, researchers study racial rather than socioeconomic diversity. I limited the sample to two races, white and black, in order to have enough women of each race to make significant comparisons and conclusions. As researchers (for example, Huddleston et al. 2010) have noted, however, differences in infertility experiences exist among other races and ethnicities as well. For example, Hispanic women use ARTs less frequently than do white women (Feinberg et al. 2007). Such differences call for more in-depth analyses that examine the social and cultural bases of such differences.

In comparing black and white women of low SES in this study, however, I found few instances of race differences in the experiences of infertility. There were far more similarities between black and white women of low SES than between the women belonging to different socioeconomic groups. There are many explanations for such trends, but perhaps most significant is that infertility is a *medicalized* phenomenon, and thus access to its treatment is at the core of its construction and understanding. In turn, class, not race, takes center stage because economic components (for example, insurance and scheduling) both structurally and ideologically primarily drive access to medicine. That is definitely not to say, however, that race does not play a significant role in shaping an individual's experience of infertility. As I noted throughout the book, less disclosure of personal issues, lower marital rates, and negative attitudes toward medicine are several key differences between white women and black women.

In addition to race, experiences differ among sexualities as well. By chance, the sample was not diverse with respect to sexual orientation with only one participant self-identifying as lesbian. Exploring infertility among women with different sexual identities would expose differences in not only involuntary childlessness but also family formation more generally. Unlike their heterosexual counterparts, lesbian couples' procreation is "forced" to be planned and medicalized; how this alters experiences needs further examination.

Why These Findings Matter

Why are these findings important? Why do they matter? At the most basic level, understanding the class dynamics of infertility challenges the conventional wisdom about *who* becomes infertile and *what* the experience of infertility is. The findings tell us that infertility occurs among all types of women and goes beyond the doctor's office. Infertility is a social process, influenced by the context in which one lives, including the class, race, and gendered practices and messages about infertility women receive. Thus, overcoming such stereotypes allows us to not only better understand infertility itself, but it also reveals the larger social factors at play, including reproduction, motherhood, and medicine.

The women's stories reveal the deeply embedded classist ideas about who should reproduce. In fact, the women themselves, both low and high SES, employ class-based ideologies when talking about infertility and reproduction. All participants reify the notion that money is necessary to be a good mother by comparing themselves to bad mothers who have children "they cannot afford." Similarly, the institutional practices of medicine, such as appointment scheduling, insurance coverage, and differential treatment of affluent and poor patients, reflect a two-class system of health care that rations treatment according to the ability to pay. These practices, attuned to the needs and schedules of affluent patients, make infertility treatment accessible to wealthy women while imposing insurmountable barriers that deter women of low SES from seeking medical care. The institutional practices of medicine are therefore consistent with classist notions of what groups should reproduce by providing infertility treatment to women of high SES while excluding women of low SES from receiving services. In other words, comparing class experiences of infertility demonstrates the continued presence of "stratified reproduction" in America.

Once we recognize the deep and pervasive inequality that characterizes the way our society defines and treats reproduction, it becomes possible to envision alternative possibilities. Most current efforts to reduce disparities in infertility focus on increasing access to health insurance and medical treatment. But understanding infertility as a social, rather than merely a medical, issue suggests that it is necessary yet insufficient to focus exclusively on access to medical treatment; we must begin resolving ideological issues as well. As one researcher notes, resolving disparities in infertility will require "more than simply a call for access to choices not of our own making" (Steinberg 1997, 45). Without reviewing the ideological notions of class-based motherhood and the classist structure of medicine, inequalities in the provision of infertility treatments will remain. Beyond lobbying for comprehensive insurance coverage of infertility treatments, we also need to critically examine the provision of infertility treatment to develop context-appropriate solutions.

Focusing exclusively on medical solutions, however, limits our understanding of the experiences of infertility. Doing so fails to recognize variation in infertility experiences and also reinforces the social control, social norms, and biomedical understanding surrounding the medicalization of infertility (Donchin 1996). While treatment disparities need to be resolved, we must also recognize experiences in which nonmedical, folk methods are employed. Future research must avoid privileging biomedical solutions (Becker et al. 2006) and instead step outside medicalized infertility to acknowledge experiences that are not medically resolved, yet still "successfully" overcome.

This study, then, suggests that we need to broaden our thinking about infertility to address the needs of the diverse women who encounter the problem. In addition, the findings suggest that we need to more broadly reconsider and reexamine reproductive policy. Family planning programs, adoption procedures, and welfare regulations are all based on mainstream understandings of who should reproduce and who should have children. For instance, many family planning programs target low-income neighborhoods in an effort to prevent unintended pregnancies, but, as the findings reveal, our understanding of pregnancy intent is based on higher-class notions of the concept. For this reason, the pregnancies of some women of low SES who, like the women in this study, clearly want to become pregnant, may be miscategorized as unintentional, and we may systematically overestimate the prevalence of unintended pregnancies. Without an accurate estimate of the scope of the problem, our interventions may be misguided. Researchers have assessed that unintended pregnancies publicly cost approximately $11 billion (Sonfield et al. 2011). Such costs may be minimized if we have a more precise estimate of the unmet need for contraception and more efficiently use resources in programs that prevent pregnancies that are truly unintentional.

In her interview, Angie, a black woman of low SES, contended that adoption agencies "pick and prod" into your life to "judge" whether you will be an adequate and appropriate parent. That scrutiny coupled with the exorbitant cost of adopting a child causes many women of low SES to avoid adoption as a solution to their childlessness. In addition to such explicit exclusionary measures, adoption procedures implicitly exclude women of low SES and other marginalized mothers from adopting through restrictions, such as making adoption only available to married couples. Based on a heteronormative notion of a "normal" family, these policies not only exclude single women and lesbian women from adopting, but they also implicitly and unconsciously remove many black women from consideration because fewer (low SES) black women marry than their white counterparts. The findings bring such practices to light, but they also reveal the need and desire to adopt among the groups that are excluded. Thus, efforts should be made to develop more inclusive adoption policies that are less bureaucratic than the "Social Security" application that Angie equates them to and more in line with the needs and desires of all potential adoptive parents.

Most of this book reveals the trials and tribulations of infertility. Concentrating only on the negative aspects of infertility, however, can itself result in negative consequences. Portraying infertility as "bad" reinforces the normality of motherhood and children. In other words, it reifies the notion that women should not be childless and, in turn, "mandates motherhood." We need to remember women such as Roberta, who focused on the positive aspects of her childlessness, such as time to devote to school and travel, and was thus able to "overcome" its negative aspects. In revealing such triumphant stories, the findings begin to lend validity to the idea that, for some women, childlessness as a viable option calls into question norms and values that equate motherhood with health and normalcy. Readjusting the emphasis also helps to remove infertility from the realm of medicine by showing solutions to childlessness other than just trying to become pregnant. Because it is focused exclusively on producing a biological child, medicine often overshadows life beyond infertility and childlessness. Listening to the voices of the women of low SES in this study, however, reminds us that biological parenthood is not the only way to achieve motherhood and that motherhood is not the only route to health and fulfillment.

This book allows us to conceive of infertility in a new light. Infertility is not merely a disease to be treated or an ailment that affects only the higher classes. As psychologists Miriam Ulrich and Ann Weatherall (2000, 334) have explained, "infertility provides a lens for viewing motherhood and the disciplinary power of discourses about motherhood." Indeed, examining the class aspects of infertility exposes how reproduction is both a private and public phenomenon. It allows us to go beyond the familial and medical contexts in which it is typically studied to examine its cultural and social dimensions as well (Clarke 1998). By placing stories such as Angie's alongside stories like those of Sarah, we can "re-conceive" infertility and the social powers that shape it.

Appendix: Methodology

The Participants

Between 2008 and 2010, I interviewed sixty-three women about their experiences of infertility. To better understand the socioeconomic components of the experience, I recruited women of both high and low SES. In particular, I oversampled economically disadvantaged women because their experiences are largely absent from both popular and academic discourse. Additionally, in an effort to not generalize by class, I recruited both black and white women to participate in the study. As stated in my introduction, however, gaining such diversity in the high SES group was difficult despite my efforts. I undertook targeted recruitment of black women of high SES by advertising at black sororities, African American churches, predominantly black civic organizations, and in other research projects studying that population. Despite such efforts, I only recruited three black participants of high SES. Given such small numbers, I eliminated their interviews from the analysis. I also removed two additional interviews with women that identified as Latina. Thus, the analyses in this book are based on fifty-eight in-depth, semistructured interviews with three groups of women: twenty white low SES women, twenty-one black low SES women, and seventeen white women of high SES.

In addition to race and class, the participants had to be between the ages of eighteen and forty-four. This age range reflects that of the participants in the National Survey of Family Growth (NSFG), the largest national survey examining fertility. Limiting the ages to such childbearing years also restricts participants to those who are currently infertile or have recently experienced infertility. The present study is also limited to women who have ever experienced involuntary childlessness for at least one year due to the inability to conceive or carry a child to term. Phrasing recruitment in this way allowed me to interview women who met the medical definition of infertility, while not medicalizing the condition or labeling the women as infertile. Some women might not identify as infertile and may view it as a stigmatizing label. Moreover, one of my main goals at the outset was to see if the participants conceived of their infertility as a medical condition so I did not want to preemptively medicalize it through recruitment. It may seem counterintuitive that I use the term "infertility" throughout the book given this logic. I do so, however, to converse with current literature as well as employ a term that is commonly recognized by the general public.

I recruited participants through posting flyers, snowball sampling, and online advertising. I posted flyers at public venues, such as libraries and grocery stores. I also posted them at places affiliated with low-income individuals, in particular, such as homeless shelters, food banks, laundromats, and public housing sites. Additionally, I posted an advertisement on the web-based classified advertising site craigslist.org. The advertisement was identical to the flyer and yielded about the same number of participants. To ensure that online advertising did not recruit a different type of person, I compared analyses on a few key themes and did not find any variations from women recruited via flyers and other mechanisms. I only recruited one participant by word of mouth who had heard about the study through an acquaintance. It is important to note that I did not recruit participants from medical clinics. I did not want to limit the analyses to those who had already medicalized the condition or to those who sought only medical treatment for infertility rather than alternatives.

To group the women by economic status, I first had to define what I meant by such a concept. "Social class" is an ambiguous term, in both popular usage and academic parlance. The specific discipline to which I claim membership, sociology, cannot even agree on its definition (Lareau 2008). This is at least in part because class encompasses many dimensions of an individual's life: income, occupation, educational level, family background, family size, and so on. Given the sheer number of factors involved, it is no wonder that scholars find it so difficult to agree on how it should be measured, but the very complexity and ambiguity of the concept of class should not deter us from studying it. Class is an important and influential aspect of life experiences, and researchers have found that it plays a particularly significant role in shaping family structure (Lareau 2003). Thus, given that I was not going to shy away from studying social class due to its complexity, I had to develop a way to categorize participants by social class that, I believe, satisfies both objective and subjective definitions of the concept. Rather than the term "class," however, I chose to use the phrase "socioeconomic status" when referring to the participants for a variety of reasons. First, socioeconomic status encompasses the numerous economic *and* social facets of class position that are present in the women's everyday lives, such as occupation, education, family background, and income. It also represents the hierarchical ranking and relationships among socioeconomic strata in society (Krieger, Williams, and Moss 1997). Second, I wanted to avoid using the pejorative phrase "lower-class" and felt that low socioeconomic status better encompassed and represented the women in the group.

I looked at a variety of factors to determine the participants' SES group. Before being interviewed, participants completed a demographic questionnaire in which I asked several questions, many of which were to determine a woman's SES. These included questions about the woman's occupation and education along with her partner's, her parents' education, household income, household size, and a subjective question about whether she viewed her income as adequate.

As a starting point, I began grouping women according to their household incomes. Not only is income one of the three primary variables encompassed in the concept of socioeconomic status (in addition to occupation and education), but it is also the variable upon which women are explicitly excluded from infertility treatments due to the cost of medical treatment and its connection to insurance. Income, however, is a highly sensitive topic that participants may not fully disclose. Therefore, I used the other indicators of SES, including the occupation and educational attainment of the participants and their households to verify the income categorization and determine the final groupings of participants. In the majority of cases, these variables, taken together, corresponded to income. For those who did not clearly fall into a particular SES group, primarily due to a disjuncture between education and income, I based the category on a variety of factors. For instance, I categorized a social worker who earns $35,000 annually and whose parents are professors as high SES; whereas I classified a factory worker who earns $50,000 a year, who did not graduate high school, and whose parents did not graduate as low SES. These women, whose SES resisted easy classification, were the exception rather than the rule: grouping women according to income typically resulted in consistency across income, education, and occupation. Defining socioeconomic status in this way and based on the inductive division of the findings resulted in two overarching SES groups: low SES, which, in terms of class, includes both poor and working-class women, and high SES, which includes both middle-class and upper-middle-class women.

The findings themselves lead to this binary socioeconomic division. Despite class variation in each SES group, the experiences of poor and working-class women, for example, were very similar, as were those of the middle- and upper-middle-class women, a realization that echoed findings from previous studies on class (for example, Blum 1999 and Lareau 2003). Throughout the book I highlight the few instances where variation did occur (for example, more middle-class women adopt than do upper-middle-class women).

Of high SES women 76 percent were college educated, whereas only 5 percent of women in the low SES groups had a college degree. Women of high SES reported an average annual household income of $90,000 compared to $30,000 reported by white women of low SES and $10,000 reported by black women of low SES. All high SES women were covered by private health insurance; 55 percent of white women of low SES were, and only one-third of black women of low SES received such benefit. On average, the women were in their early thirties, with black low SES women slightly younger (twenty-nine years) than the white women of the other SES groups (low SES: thirty-three years; high SES: thirty-five years). All women of high SES were married compared to only 19 percent of black women of low SES and 60 percent of white women of low SES.

Interviewing

Immediately after posting flyers, the phone began to ring, and I started interviewing. I conducted all interviews in person. They were semistructured in that I had an interview guide, but I asked questions based on the participants' responses and thus, added, altered, and removed some questions based on the conversations. All interviews covered the entire infertility journey, beginning with the respondent's family background, and then walking through life before infertility, recognizing childbearing difficulties, living with infertility, and then trying to resolve and cope with infertility. Interviews lasted, on average, 90 minutes, with a range between

30 and 150 minutes. I typically suggested interviewing in study rooms of public libraries, but I ultimately let the participant decide the space. Thus, the majority of interviews were at libraries, but some were held at different locations (for example, participant's home, park, or restaurant). I gave all participants a $10 grocery store gift card after completing the interview.

The quotes I selected for the book represent the most illustrative examples from the interview transcripts. I was acutely aware, however, of highlighting the diversity of the sample and diligently tried to avoid repetitively using a handful of the most prolific interviews. As a result, fifty-two of the fifty-eight eligible interview participants are represented in these pages.

One advantage of this research is the diversity of its participants, in turn exposing infertility as a diverse process. With such an advantage, however, come some methodological limitations. As the sole researcher on this project, my numerous identities (that is, a white, educated, middle-class woman and a researcher) were shared by only a handful of the participants. For this reason, it was important for me to consider how my identities may have affected the interview or the study's findings.

A common method for addressing demographic differences between researcher and researched is to eliminate those differences altogether though researcher-subject concordance—that is, by "matching" the participant with an interviewer that has similar characteristics, typically along one dimension (for example, race). Primarily used in survey and quantitative research, this strategy is said to offer several advantages: when researcher and subject share a common culture, researchers are arguably better able to understand and interpret participants' perspectives, and participants are more likely to trust and speak freely to researchers with similar characteristics. For these reasons, proponents argue that concordance leads to a deeper conversation in the interview and can enhance the credibility of the study's findings and conclusions.

Despite these advantages, there are also cogent arguments against researcher-subject concordance. First, matching interviewer and subject along a certain dimension assumes that there is a single truth that can only be attained between individuals sharing particular traits. As sociologist Yasmin Gunaratnam (2009, 88) has argued, this assumption "is based upon a logic of commonality as emotional and ethical unity, where race, ethnicity, and/or culture are imagined as imbuing research interactions with levels of communication, trust, and care that precede the research relationships themselves." I believe that experiences produce several accounts–none of which is superior, and all are meaningful and interesting in their own right. For instance, in a study on foster parents (a topic similar to infertility) a researcher found that black participants were particularly eager to share their perspective with white interviewers and, in fact, revealed more to them. Therefore, rather than serving as a barrier to communication, difference between researcher and researched can provoke conversation, particularly when studying marginalized groups. Second, matching the characteristics of interviewer and respondent is based on the questionable a priori assumption that one social signifier, such as race, will dominate other dimensions of difference, such as gender or class.

Ultimately, differences between researcher and researched do make a difference to a study's findings and conclusions. Yasmin Gunaratnam (2009, 81) suggests, however, that "the difference that our difference can make in researching a sensitive topic such as infertility is multilayered and multisided." Because of the pragmatic constraints of time and money as well as the intellectual reasons I just mentioned, I used techniques other than interviewer matching to deal with difference. I designed some interview questions to explicitly tease out race differences in infertility experiences. I also developed techniques and skills to gain participants' trust. Intent listening, eye contact, engagement with the participant, and easing into the topic of infertility with broad, general questions helped create a comfortable environment for the respondents so that our differences did not preclude a relaxed, in-depth conversation.

While it is likely that my identities shaped what the participants told me, there is reason to believe that their stories were not sufficiently different to distort the research findings. My interviews were of similar length, and no participant ever inquired about my race or educational background and their influences on our interaction. Instead, several participants thanked me for the opportunity to talk, as many had never discussed their fertility issues with anyone else. Indeed, similar to Lorraine Culley and her colleagues' (2007) research of infertility among South Asian women, my research participants may have identified my status as "expert" rather than my ethnicity as the salient social identity. My affiliation with a university seemed to reassure participants of my trustworthiness and knowledge surrounding infertility and their experiences. Because infertility is a medicalized phenomenon, it is automatically associated with talking to "objective" others, such as doctors, about the condition. Also, because infertility is gendered or considered a woman's issue, my identity as a woman may have trumped my race and class positions and may have facilitated my conversations with participants. It is, of course, impossible to know how my identities affected participants in the study. For this reason, I view this project as an exploratory study of class and infertility and invite researchers of different backgrounds to study this subject.

Notes

Introduction: Conceiving Infertility

1. Higher rates of infertility among women of low SES and black women are due to class- and race-specific trends, such as a higher prevalence of sexually transmitted infections among their populations (Chandra et al. 2005).
2. The Patient Protection and Affordable Care Act (that is, "Obamacare") enacted on March 23, 2010, does not include specific provisions for or expansion of medical benefits for infertility care.
3. An ART cycle typically includes three phases: (1) ovarian simulation phase where the eggs are developed; (2) ART phase in which the specific procedure, for example, intrauterine insemination (IUI), in vitro fertilization (IVF), or frozen embryo transfer, occurs; and (3) the luteal phase in which implantation of the embryo occurs, resulting in a pregnancy.
4. Across ages, 30 percent is the average success rate. Success rates vary according to age: 41.5% (< 35 years); 31.9% (35–37); 22.1% (38–40); 12.4% (41–42); 5% (43–44), 1% (> 44).
5. But the open criteria also have limitations. First, "recall bias," or skewing your story due to the inability to remember all the details, might be of concern for those who experienced infertility many years ago. Second, there may be some misalignment between the women's current demographic characteristics (for example, marital status, household income) collected at time of interview and those characteristics during their experiences of infertility. Such limitations, however, were only minimally present, if at all, in this study.
6. In terms of demographic changes through time, much of that was resolved within the interview. For instance, when discussing the relationship between marital status and infertility, I phrased the question(s) to refer to the time of the infertile experience (for example, to what extent and how did your childbearing difficulty impact your relationship?). Further, for variables, such as social class, I took extra care to ensure that such demographics were consistent through time. For example, the compilation of variables comprising the class categories not only provided a thorough definition of class, but it also allowed me to examine the participants' past class standing as evinced by their parents' education and then compare it to their current status. Through such comparison, I found no evidence that class status changed for any of the participants.

5. "Whatever Gets Me to the End Point": Resolving Infertility

Portions of this chapter were previously published in "'It's way out of my league': Low-Income Women's Experiences of Medicalized Infertility," *Gender & Society* 23 (5) (2009); and "Beyond (Financial) Accessibility: Inequalities within the Medicalization of Infertility," *Sociology of Health & Illness* 32 (4) (2010).

6. "So What Can You Do?": Coping with infertility

Portions of this chapter have been previously published in "'It's way out of my league': Low-Income Women's Experiences of Medicalized Infertility," *Gender & Society* 23 (5) (2009) and "Beyond (Financial) Accessibility: Inequalities within the Medicalization of Infertility," *Sociology of Health & Illness* 32 (4) (2010).

References

Abramovitz, Mimi. 1995. "From Tenement Class to Dangerous Class to Underclass: Blaming Women for Social Problems." In *Feminist Practice in the 21ˢᵗ Century,* edited by Nan van den Bergh, 211–231. Washington, DC: National Association of Social Workers.

American Society for Reproductive Medicine. 2013a. "State Infertility Insurance Laws." Accessed April 26. http://www.asrm.org/insurance.aspx.

———. 2013b. "Is In Vitro Fertilization Expensive?" Accessed May 31. http://www.asrm.org/detail.aspx?id=3023.

Anspach, Renee. 1993. "The Language of Case Presentation." In *The Sociology of Health and Illness: Critical Perspectives,* edited by Peter Conrad, 320–338. New York: Worth Publishers.

Arendell, Terry. 2000. "Conceiving and Investigating Motherhood: The Decade's Scholarship." *Journal of Marriage and Family* 62: 1192–1207.

Augustine, Jennifer March, Timothy Nelson, and Kathryn Edin. 2009. "Why Do Poor Men Have Children? Fertility Intentions among Low-income Unmarried U.S. Fathers." *Annals of the American Academy of Political and Social Science* 624: 99–117.

Baker, Phyllis L., and Amy Carson. 1999. "'I Take Care of my Kids': Mothering Practices of Substance-Abusing Women." *Gender & Society* 13: 347–363.

Barker, Kristin K. 2008. "Electronic Support Groups, Patient-Consumers, and Medicalization: The Case of Contested Illness." *Journal of Health and Social Behavior* 49: 20–36.

Barrett, Geraldine, and Kaye Wellings. 2002. "What Is a 'Planned' Pregnancy? Empirical Data from a British Study." *Social Science & Medicine* 55: 545–557.

Bates, G. William, and Susanne R. Bates. 1996. "Infertility Services in a Managed Care Environment." *Current Opinion in Obstetrics and Gynecology* 8: 300–304.

Becker, Gay. 2000. *The Elusive Embryo: How Women and Men Approach New Reproductive Technologies.* Berkeley: University of California Press.

Becker, Gay, Martha Castrillo, Rebecca Jackson, and Robert D. Nachtigall. 2006. "Infertility among Low-income Latinos." *Fertility and Sterility* 85: 882–887.

Becker, Gay, and Robert D. Nachtigall. 1992. "Eager for Medicalisation: The Social Production of Infertility as a Disease." *Sociology of Health & Illness* 14: 456–471.

Bell, Ann V. 2009. "'It's way out of my league': Low-Income Women's Experiences of Medicalized Infertility." *Gender & Society* 23: 688–709.

———. 2010. "Beyond (Financial) Accessibility: Inequalities within the Medicalization of Infertility." *Sociology of Health & Illness* 32: 631–646.

Berry, Mary Frances. 1993. *The Politics of Parenthood: Child Care, Women's Rights, and the Myth of the Good Mother.* New York: Penguin Books.

Bhalla, Ajit, and Frederic Lapeyre. 1997. "Social Exclusion: Towards an Analytical and Operational Framework." *Development and Change* 28: 413–433.

Bitler, Marianne, and Lucie Schmidt. 2006. "Health Disparities and Infertility: Impacts of State-Level Insurance Mandates." *Fertility and Sterility* 85: 858–865.

———. 2012. "Utilization of Infertility Treatments: The Effects of Insurance Mandates." *Demography* 49: 125–149.

Blum, Linda M. 1999. *At the Breast: Ideologies of Breastfeeding and Motherhood in the Contemporary United States.* Boston: Beacon Press.

Blum, Linda, and Theresa Deussen. 1996. "Negotiating Independent Motherhood: Working-Class African American Women Talk about Marriage and Motherhood." *Gender & Society* 10: 199–211.

Bolam, Bruce, Darrin Hodgetts, Kerry Chamberlain, Simon Murphy, and Kate Gleeson. 2003. "'Just do it': An Analysis of Accounts of Control over Health amongst Lower Socioeconomic Status Groups." *Critical Public Health* 13: 15–31.

Breheny, Mary, and Christine Stephens. 2007. "Irreconcilable Differences: Health Professionals' Constructions of Adolescence and Motherhood." *Social Science & Medicine* 64: 112–124.

Brubaker, Sarah Jane. 2007. "Denied, Embracing, and Resisting Medicalization: African-American Teen Mothers' Perceptions of Formal Pregnancy and Childbirth Care." *Gender & Society* 21: 528–552.

Brubaker, Sarah Jane, and Christie Wright. 2006. "Identity Transformation and Family Caregiving: Narratives of African American Teen Mothers." *Journal of Marriage & Family* 68: 1214–1228.

Burton, Linda M. 1990. "Teenage Childbearing as an Alternative Lifecourse Strategy in Multigenerational Black Families." *Human Nature* 1: 123–143.

Ceballo, Rosario. 1999. "'The Only Black Woman Walking the Face of the Earth Who Cannot Have a Baby': Two Women's Stories." In *Women's Untold Stories: Breaking Silence, Talking Back, Voicing Complexity,* edited by Mary Romero and Abigail J. Stewart, 3–19. New York: Routledge.

Centers for Disease Control and Prevention. 2013a. Assisted Reproductive Technology. Accessed June 3. http://www.cdc.gov/art/

———. 2013b. National ART Success Rates. Accessed June 3. http://apps.nccd.cdc.gov/art/Apps/NationalSummaryReport.aspx

Chandra, Anjani, Casey E. Copen, and Elizabeth Hervey Stephen. 2013. "Infertility and Impaired Fecundity in the United States, 1982–2010: Data from the National Survey of Family Growth." National Center for Health Statistics. *Vital Health Statistics,* 67.

Chandra, Anjani, Gladys M. Martinez, William D. Mosher, Joyce C. Abma, and Jo Jones. 2005. "Fertility, Family Planning, and Reproductive Health of U.S. Women: Data from the 2002 National Survey of Family Growth." National Center for Health Statistics. *Vital Health Statistics,* 23.

Chandra, Anjani, Elizabeth Hervey Stephen, and Rosalind Berkowitz King. 2013. "Infertility Service Use among Fertility-Impaired Women in the United States: 1995–2010." Paper presented to the Population Association of America Annual Meeting, April 11–13, New Orleans, Louisiana. http://paa2013.princeton.edu/papers/130548.

Chodorow, Nancy. 1978. *The Reproduction of Mothering.* Berkeley: University of California Press.

Clarke, Adele E. 1998. *Disciplining Reproduction: Modernity, American Life Sciences, and "the Problems of Sex."* Berkeley: University of California Press.

Colen, Shellee. 1986. "'With Respect and Feelings': Voices of West Indian Child Care and Domestic Workers in New York City." In *All American Women: Lives That Divide, Ties That Bind,* edited by Johnetta B. Cole, 46–70. New York: Free Press.

Collins, Patricia Hill. 1990. *Black Feminist Thought: Knowledge, Consciousness, and the Politics of Empowerment.* New York: Routledge.

———. 1994. "Shifting the Center: Race, Class, and Feminist Theorizing about Motherhood." In *Mothering: Ideology, Experience, and Agency,* edited by Evelyn Nakano Glenn, Grace Chang, and Linda Rennie Forcey, 45–66. New York: Routledge.

Connolly, Deborah. 2000. "Mythical Mothers and Dichotomies of Good and Evil: Homeless Mothers in the United States." In *Ideologies and Technologies of Motherhood,* edited by Helena Ragone and France Winddance Twine, 263–294. New York: Routledge.

Conrad, Peter. 1990. "Qualitative Research on Chronic Illness: A Commentary on Method and Conceptual Development." *Social Science & Medicine* 30: 1257–1263.

Conrad, Peter, and Valerie Leiter. 2004. "Medicalization, Markets and Consumers." *Journal of Health and Social Behavior* 45: 158–176.

Cooey, Paula M. 1999. "'Ordinary Mother' as Oxymoron: The Collusion of Theology, Theory, and Politics in the Undermining of Mothers." In *Mother Troubles: Rethinking Contemporary Maternal Dilemmas,* edited by Julia E. Hanigsberg and Sara Ruddick, 229–249. Boston: Beacon Press.

Culley, Lorraine. 2009. "Dominant Narratives and Excluded Voices: Research on Ethnic Differences in Access to Assisted Conception in More Developed Societies." In *Marginalized Reproduction: Ethnicity, Infertility, and Reproductive Technologies,* edited by Lorraine Culley, Nicky Hudson, and Floor van Rooij, 17–33. London: Earthscan Publishers.

Culley, Lorraine, Nicky Hudson, and Frances Rapport. 2007. "Using Focus Groups with Minority Ethnic Communities: Researching Infertility in British South Asian Communities." *Qualitative Health Research* 17: 102–112.

Cussins, Charis. 1998. "Producing Reproduction: Techniques of Normalization and Naturalization in Infertility Clinics." In *Reproducing Reproduction: Kinship, Power, and Technological Innovation,* edited by Sarah Franklin and Helena Ragone, 66–101. Philadelphia: University of Pennsylvania Press.

Davidson, Rosemary, Jenny Kitzinger, and Kate Hunt. 2006. "The Wealthy Get Healthy, the Poor Get Poorly? Lay Perceptions of Health Inequalities." *Social Science & Medicine* 62: 2171–2182.

De Lacey, Sheryl. 2002. "IVF as Lottery or Investment: Contesting Metaphors in Discourses of Infertility." *Nursing Inquiry* 9: 43–51.

Dillaway, Heather, and Sarah Jane Brubaker. 2006. "Intersectionality and Childbirth: How Women from Different Social Locations Discuss Epidural Use." *Race, Gender & Class* 13: 16–42.

Donchin, Anne. 1996. "Feminist Critiques of New Fertility Technologies: Implications for Social Policy." *Journal of Medicine & Philosophy* 21: 475–498.

Earle, Sarah, and Gayle Letherby. 2003. "Introducing Gender, Identity, and Reproduction." In *Gender, Identity, and Reproduction: Social Perspectives,* edited by Sarah Earle and Gayle Letherby, 1–12. New York: Palgrave Macmillan.

Edin, Kathryn, and Maria Kefalas. 2005. *Promises I Can Keep: Why Poor Women Put Motherhood Before Marriage.* Berkeley: University of California Press.

Ehrenreich, Barbara, and Deirdre English. 1979. *For Her Own Good: 150 Years of the Experts' Advice to Women.* New York: Anchor Books.

Ellison, Christopher G., Jason D. Boardman, David R. Williams, and James S. Jackson. 2001. "Religious Involvement, Stress, and Mental Health: Findings from the 1995 Detroit Area Study." *Social Forces* 80: 215–249.

Evans, Donald. 1995. "Infertility and the NHS: Purchasers Should Avoid the Moral High Ground." *British Medical Journal* 311: 1586–1587.

Feinberg, Eve C., Frederick W. Larsen, Robert M. Wah, Ruben J. Alvergo, and Alicia Y. Armstrong. 2007. "Economics May Not Explain Hispanic Underutilization of Assisted Reproductive Technology Services." *Fertility and Sterility* 88: 1439–1441.

Fisher, Sue. 1986. *In the Patient's Best Interest: Women and the Politics of Medical Decisions.* New Brunswick, NJ: Rutgers University Press.

Foucault, Michel. 1975. *Birth of the Clinic: An Archaeology of Medical Perception.* New York: Vintage.

Franklin, Sarah. 1992. "Contested Conceptions: A Cultural Account of Assisted Reproduction." PhD diss., University of Birmingham, England.

———. 2013. *Biological Relatives: IVF, Stem Cells, and the Future of Kinship.* Durham, NC: Duke University Press.

Freidson, Eliot. 1960. "Client Control and Medical Practice." *American Journal of Sociology* 65: 374–382.

———. 1972. *Profession of Medicine.* New York: Dodd-Mead.

Furstenberg, Frank F. 1987. "Race Differences in Teenage Sexuality, Pregnancy, and Adolescent Childbearing." *The Milbank Quarterly* 65: 381–403.

Gamble, Vanessa Northington. 1997. "Under the Shadow of Tuskegee: African Americans and Health Care." *American Journal of Public Health* 87: 1773–1778.

Ganong, Lawrence H., and Marilyn Coleman. 1995. "The Content of Mother Stereotypes." *Sex Roles* 32: 495–512.

Geertz, Clifford. 1973. *The Interpretation of Cultures.* New York: Basic Books.

Ginsburg, Faye, and Rayna Rapp. 1991. "The Politics of Reproduction." *Annual Review of Anthropology* 20: 311–343.

Glenn, Evelyn Nakano. 1994. "Social Constructions of Mothering: A Thematic Overview." In *Mothering: Ideology, Experience, and Agency,* edited by Evelyn Nakano Glenn, Grace Chang, and Linda Rennie Forcey, 1–32. New York: Routledge.

———. 2010. *Forced to Care: Coercion and Caregiving in America.* Cambridge, MA: Harvard University Press.

Gordon, Linda. 2002. *The Moral Property of Women: A History of Birth Control Politics in America.* Urbana: University of Illinois Press.

Greil, Arthur L. 1991. *Not Yet Pregnant: Infertile Couples in Contemporary America.* New Brunswick, NJ: Rutgers University Press.

———. 1997. "Infertility and Psychological Distress: A Critical Review of the Literature." *Social Science & Medicine* 45: 1679–1704.

Greil, Arthur L., Thomas A. Leitko, and Karen L. Porter. 1988. "Infertility: His and Hers." *Gender & Society* 2: 172–199.

Greil, Arthur L., and Julia McQuillan. 2010. "'Trying' Times: Medicalization, Intent, and Ambiguity in the Definition of Infertility." *Medical Anthropology Quarterly* 24: 137–156.

Greil, Arthur L., Julia McQuillan, Michele Lowry, and Karina M. Shreffler. 2011a. "Infertility Treatment and Fertility-Specific Distress: A Longitudinal Analysis of a Population-based Sample of U.S. Women." *Social Science and Medicine* 73: 87–94.

Greil, Arthur L., Julia McQuillan, Karina M. Shreffler, Katherine M. Johnson, and Kathleen Slauson-Blevins. 2011b. "Race-Ethnicity and Medical Services for Infertility Stratified Reproduction in a Population-based Sample of U.S. Women." *Journal of Health and Social Behavior* 52: 493–509.

Greil, Arthur L., Julia McQuillan, and Kathleen Slauson-Blevins. 2011. "The Social Construction of Infertility." *Sociology Compass* 5: 736–746.

Greil, Arthur L., Kathleen Slauson-Blevins, and Julia McQuillan. 2010. "The Experience of Infertility: A Review of Recent Literature." *Sociology of Health & Illness* 32: 1–23.

Gunaratnam, Yasmin. 2009. "What Difference Does Our Difference Make in Researching Infertility?" In *Marginalized Reproduction: Ethnicity, Infertility, and Reproductive Technologies,* edited by Lorraine Culley, Nicky Hudson, and Floor van Rooij, 80–94. London: Earthscan Publishers.

Harding, David J. 2007. "Cultural Context, Sexual Behavior, and Romantic Relationships in Disadvantaged Neighborhoods." *American Sociological Review* 72: 341–364.

Hasenfeld, Yeheskel. 2010. "The Attributes of Human Service Organizations." In *Human Services as Complex Organizations,* edited by Yeheskel Hasenfeld, 9–32. Newbury Park, CA: Sage Publications.

Hays, Sharon. 1996. *The Cultural Contradictions of Motherhood.* New Haven: Yale University Press.

Heitman, Elizabeth. 1995. "Infertility as a Public Health Problem: Why Assisted Reproductive Technologies Are Not the Answer." *Stanford Law & Policy Review* 6: 89–102.

Henifin, Mary S. 1993. "New Reproductive Technologies: Equity and Access to Reproductive Health Care." *Journal of Social Issues* 49: 61–74.

Hennessy, Judith. 2009. "Morality and Work-Family Conflict in the Lives of Poor and Low-Income Women." *Sociological Quarterly* 50: 557–580.

Hill, Shirley A. 1994. "Motherhood and the Obfuscation of Medical Knowledge: The Case of Sickle Cell Disease." *Gender & Society* 8: 29–47.

———. 2004. *Black Intimacies: A Gender Perspective on Families and Relationships.* New York: Rowman & Littlefield Publishers.

———. 2009. "Cultural Images and the Health of African American Women." *Gender & Society* 23: 733–746.

Hondagneu-Sotelo, Pierrette, and Ernestine Avila. 1997. "'I'm Here, but I'm There': The Meanings of Latina Transnational Motherhood." *Gender & Society* 11: 548–571.

Huddleston, Heather G., Marcelle I. Cedars, Sae H. Sohn, Linda C. Giudice, and Victor Y. Fujimoto. 2010. "Racial and Ethnic Disparities in Reproductive Endocrinology and Infertility." *American Journal of Obstetrics & Gynecology* 202: 413–419.

Inhorn, Marcia, Rosario Ceballo, and Robert Nachtigall. 2009. "Marginalized, Invisible, and Unwanted: American Minority Struggles with Infertility and Assisted Conception." In *Marginalized Reproduction: Ethnicity, Infertility, and Assisted Conception,* edited by Lorraine Culley, Nicky Hudson, and Floor van Rooij, 181–198. London: Earthscan Publishers.

Jain, Tarun. 2006. "Socioeconomic and Racial Disparities among Infertility Patients Seeking Care." *Fertility & Sterility* 85: 876–881.

Jain, Tarun, and Mark D. Hornstein. 2005. "Disparities in Access to Infertility Services in a State with Mandated Insurance Coverage." *Fertility and Sterility* 84: 221–223.

Jarrett, Robin L. 1994. "Living Poor: Family Life among Single Parent, African American Women." *Social Problems* 41: 30–49.

156 • References

Jarrett, Robin L., Stephanie R. Jefferson, and Jenell N. Kelly. 2010. "Finding Community in Family: Neighborhood Effects and African American Kin Networks." Journal of Comparative Family Studies 41: 299–328.
Jones, Stephanie C., and Myra Hunter. 1996. "The Influence of Context and Discourse on Infertility Experience." Journal of Reproductive and Infant Psychology 14: 93–111.
Keeley, Bethany, Lanelle Wright, and Celeste M. Condit. 2009. "Functions of Health Fatalism: Fatalistic Talk as Face Saving, Uncertainty Management, Stress Relief, and Sense Making." Sociology of Health & Illness 31: 734–747.
Kelly, Maura. 2010. "Regulating the Reproduction and Mothering of Poor Women: The Controlling Image of the Welfare Mother in Television News Coverage of Welfare Reform." Journal of Poverty 14: 76–96.
King, Leslie, and Madonna Harrington Meyer. 1997. "The Politics of Reproductive Benefits: U.S. Insurance Coverage of Contraceptive and Infertility Treatments." Gender & Society 11: 8–30.
Kirkman, Maggie, and Doreen Rosenthal. 1999. "Representations of Reproductive Technology in Women's Narratives of Infertility." Women & Health 29: 17–35.
Klerman, Lorraine V. 2000. "The Intendedness of Pregnancy: A Concept in Transition." Maternal and Child Health Journal 4: 155–162.
Krieger, Nancy, David R. Williams, and Nancy E. Moss. 1997. "Measuring Social Class in U.S. Public Health Research: Concepts, Methodologies, and Guidelines." Annual Review of Public Health 18: 341–78.
Lareau, Annette. 2003. Unequal Childhoods: Class, Race, and Family Life. Berkeley: University of California Press.
———. 2008. "Introduction: Taking Stock of Class." In Social Class: How Does It Work?, edited by Annette Lareau and Dalton Conley, 3–24. New York: Russell Sage Foundation.
Lazarus, Ellen S. 1994. "What do Women Want?: Issues of Choice, Control, and Class in Pregnancy and Childbirth." Medical Anthropology Quarterly 8: 25–46.
Lee, Sunhwa. 2009. "Racial and Ethnic Differences in Women's Retirement Security." Journal of Women, Politics & Policy 30: 141–172.
Letherby, Gayle. 1999. "Other than Mother and Mothers as Others: The Experience of Motherhood and Non-motherhood in Relation to 'Infertility' and 'Involuntary Childlessness.'" Women's Studies International Forum 22: 359–372.
———. 2002. "Challenging Dominant Discourses: Identity and Change and the Experience of 'Infertility' and 'Involuntary Childlessness.'" Journal of Gender Studies 11: 277–288.
Litt, Jacquelyn. 1997. "American Medicine and Divided Motherhood: Three Case Studies from the 1930s and 1940s." Sociological Quarterly 38: 285–302.
Luker, Kristin. 1996. Dubious Conceptions: The Politics of Teenage Pregnancy. Cambridge, MA: Harvard University Press.
Lundquist, Jennifer Hickes, Michelle J. Budig, and Anna Curtis. 2009. "Race and Childlessness in America, 1988–2002." Journal of Marriage and Family 71: 741–755.
Marsh, Margaret S., and Wanda Ronner. 1996. The Empty Cradle: Infertility in America from Colonial Times to the Present. Baltimore: Johns Hopkins University Press.
Martin, Emily. 1990. "The Ideology of Reproduction: The Reproduction of Ideology." In Uncertain Terms: Negotiating Gender in American Culture, edited by Faye Ginsburg and Anna L. Tsing, 300–315. Boston: Beacon Press.
Martinez, Gladys M., Kimberly Daniels, and Anjani Chandra. 2012. "Fertility of Men and Women Aged 15–44 Years in the United States: National Survey of Family Growth, 2006–2010." National Health Statistics Reports 51.

Mayer, Jeffrey P. 1997. "Unintended Childbearing, Maternal Beliefs and Delay of Prenatal Care." *Birth* 24: 247–252.

McCormack, Karen. 2005. "Stratified Reproduction and Poor Women's Resistance." *Gender & Society* 19: 660–679.

McDonough, Patricia M. 1997. *Choosing Colleges: How Social Class and Schools Structure Opportunity.* Albany: State University of New York Press.

McKenna, Katelyn Y. A., and John A. Bargh. 1998. "Coming Out in the Age of the Internet: Identity 'Demarginalization' through Virtual Group Participation." *Journal of Personality and Social Psychology* 75: 681–694.

McMahon, Martha. 1995. *Engendering Motherhood: Identity and Self-transformation in Women's Lives.* New York: Guilford Press.

McQuillan, Julia, Arthur L. Greil, and Karina M. Shreffler. 2011. "Pregnancy Intentions among Women Who Do Not Try: Focusing on Women Who Are Okay Either Way." *Maternal and Child Health Journal* 15: 178–187.

Miall, Charlene E. 1986. "The Stigma of Involuntary Childlessness." *Social Problems* 33: 268–282.

———. 1989. "Reproductive Technology versus the Stigma of Involuntary Childlessness." *Social Casework: The Journal of Contemporary Social Work* 70: 43–50.

Molock, Sherry D. 1999. "Racial, Cultural, and Religious Issues in Infertility Counseling." In *Infertility Counseling: A Comprehensive Handbook for Clinicians,* edited by Linda Hammer Burns and Sharon N. Covington, 151–159. New York: Parthenon.

Moos, Merry K., Ruth Petersen, Katherine Meadows, Cathy L. Melvin, and Alison M. Spitz. 1997. "Pregnant Women's Perspectives on Intendedness of Pregnancy." *Women's Health Issues* 7: 385–392.

Nathanson, Constance A. 1991. *Dangerous Passage: The Social Control of Sexuality in Women's Adolescence.* Philadelphia: Temple University Press.

Nelson, Margaret K. 2002. "The Challenge of Self-sufficiency: Women on Welfare Redefining Independence." *Journal of Contemporary Ethnography* 31: 582–614.

Pargament, Kenneth I., and Crystal L. Park. 1995. "Merely a Defense? The Variety of Religious Means and Ends." *Journal of Social Issues* 51: 13–32.

Parry, Diana C. 2005a. "Work, Leisure, and Support Groups: An Examination of the Ways Women with Infertility Respond to Pronatalist Ideology." *Sex Roles* 53: 337–346.

———. 2005b. "Women's Experiences with Infertility: The Fluidity and Conceptualizations of 'Family.'" *Qualitative Sociology* 28: 275–291.

Quiroga, Seline S. 2007. "Blood Is Thicker than Water: Policing Donor Insemination and the Reproduction of Whiteness." *Hypatia* 22: 143–161.

Remennick, Larissa. 2000. "Childless in the Land of Imperative Motherhood: Stigma and Coping among Infertile Israeli Women." *Sex Roles* 43: 821–840.

Riessman, Catherine Kohler. 2000. "Stigma and Everyday Resistance Practices: Childless Women in South India." *Gender & Society* 14: 111–135.

Roberts, Dorothy. 1997. *Killing the Black Body: Race, Reproduction, and the Meaning of Liberty.* New York: Pantheon Books.

Rothman, Barbara Katz. 1989. *Recreating Motherhood: Ideology and Technology in a Patriarchal Society.* New York: W. W. Norton.

Ruddick, Sara. 1989. *Maternal Thinking: Toward a Politics of Peace*. Boston: Beacon Press.

Russo, Nancy F. 1976. "The Motherhood Mandate." *Journal of Social Issues* 32: 143–153.

Sandelowski, Margarete J. 1990. "Failures of Volition: Female Agency and Infertility in Historical Perspective." *Signs: Journal of Women in Culture and Society* 15: 475–499.

———.1993. *With Child in Mind: Studies of the Personal Encounter with Infertility*. Philadelphia: University of Pennsylvania Press.

Sandelowski, Margarete, and Linda Corson Jones. 1986. "Social Exchanges of Infertile Women." *Issues in Mental Health Nursing* 8: 173–189.

Schmidt, Lucie. 2007. "Effects of Infertility Insurance Mandates on Fertility." *Journal of Health Economics* 26: 431–446.

Schneider, Joseph W., and Peter Conrad. 1983. *Having Epilepsy: The Experience and Control of Illness*. Philadelphia: Temple University Press.

Scritchfield, Shirley A. 1989. "The Infertility Enterprise: IVF and the Technological Construction of Reproductive Impairments." *Research in the Sociology of Health Care* 8: 61–97.

Sewell, William H. 1992. "A Theory of Structure: Duality, Agency, and Transformation." *American Journal of Sociology* 98: 1–29.

Shattuck, Julie C., and Katherine K. Schwarz. 1991. "Walking the Line between Feminism and Infertility: Implications for Nursing, Medicine, and Patient Care." *Health Care for Women International* 12: 331–339.

Silva, Susana, and Helena Machado. 2008. "The Diagnosis of Infertility: Patients' Classification Processes and Feelings." *Medical Sociology Online* 3: 4–14.

Snow, David A., and Leon Anderson. 1987. "Identity Work among the Homeless: The Verbal Construction and Avowal of Personal Identities." *American Journal of Sociology* 92: 1336–1371.

Solinger, Rickie. 2013. *Reproductive Politics: What Everyone Needs to Know*. New York: Oxford University Press.

Sonfield, Adam, Kathryn Kost, Rachel Benson Gold, and Lawrence B. Finer. 2011. "The Public Costs of Births Resulting from Unintended Pregnancies: National and State-Level Estimates." *Perspectives on Sexual and Reproductive Health* 43: 94–102.

Spar, Debora L. 2006. *The Baby Business: How Money, Science, and Politics Drive the Commerce of Conception*. Boston: Harvard Business School Press.

Stack, Carol B. 1975. *All Our Kin: Strategies for Survival in a Black Community*. New York: Harper & Row.

Staniec, J. Farley Ordovensky, and Natalie J. Webb. 2007. "Utilization of Infertility Services: How Much Does Money Matter?" *Health Services Research* 42: 971–989.

Steinberg, Deborah L. 1997. "A Most Selective Practice: The Eugenic Logics of IVF." *Women's Studies International Forum* 20: 33–48.

Tarn, Derjung M., John Heritage, Debora A. Paterniti, Ron D. Hays, Richard L. Kravitz, and Neil S. Wenger. 2006. "Physician Communication When Prescribing New Medications." *Archives of Internal Medicine* 166: 1855–1862.

Thompson, Charis. 2005. *Making Parents: The Ontological Choreography of Reproductive Technologies*. Cambridge, MA: MIT Press.

Thorburn, Sheryl, and Laura M. Bogart. 2005. "Conspiracy Beliefs about Birth Control: Barriers to Pregnancy Prevention among African Americans of Reproductive Age." *Health Education & Behavior* 32: 474–487.

Throsby, Karen. 2004. *When IVF Fails: Feminism, Infertility, and the Negotiation of Normality*. New York: Palgrave Macmillan.

Thurer, Shari. 1994. *The Myths of Motherhood: How Culture Reinvents the Good Mother.* Boston: Houghton Mifflin.

Ulrich, Miriam, and Ann Weatherall. 2000. "Motherhood and Infertility: Viewing Motherhood through the Lens of Infertility." *Feminism & Psychology* 10: 323–336.

White, Lynn, Julia McQuillan, and Arthur L. Greil. 2006. "Explaining Disparities in Treatment Seeking: The Case of Infertility." *Fertility & Sterility* 85: 853–857.

Wilcox, Lynne S., and William D. Mosher. 1993. "Use of Infertility Services in the United States." *Obstetrics & Gynecology* 82: 122–127.

Willems, Sara, Stéphanie De Maesschalck, Myriam Deveugele, Anselme Derese, and Jan De Maeseneer. 2005. "Socio-economic Status of the Patient and Doctor–Patient Communication: Does It Make a Difference?" *Patient Education and Counseling* 56: 139–146.

Zadoroznyj, Maria. 1999. "Social Class, Social Selves, and Social Control in Childbirth." *Sociology of Health & Illness* 21: 267–289.

Zoll, Miriam. 2013. *Cracked Open: Liberty, Fertility, and the Pursuit of High-Tech Babies.* Northampton, MA: Interlink Publishing.

Index

About the Author

ANN V. BELL is an assistant professor of sociology at the University of Delaware. Her research, centering on the intersection of gender and health, specifically examines processes, inequalities, and constructions of reproductive health.

CPSIA information can be obtained at www.ICGtesting.com
Printed in the USA
BVOW07s2308160714

359023BV00004B/25/P